ALLE · [illegible] · WACH · 1842

Speech Restoration Via Voice Prostheses

Edited by I. F. Herrmann

In Collaboration with
M. Amatsu · A. D. Cheesman · C. Hammer · J. N. Hausfeld
J. L. Henley-Cohn · H. Holden · J. Lang · L. P. Löbe · H. F. Mahieu
J. J. Manni · E. Mozolewski · H. F. Nijdam · H. Rudert · A. Schauer
H. K. Schutte · R. M. Tiwari · L. Traissac · H. P. Zenner

With 95 Figures and 43 Tables

Springer-Verlag Berlin Heidelberg New York
London Paris Tokyo

Professor Dr. INGO FERDINAND HERRMANN
Universitätsklinik und Poliklinik
für Hals-, Nasen- und Ohrenkranke
im Kopfklinikum
D-8700 Würzburg/FRG

ISBN-13:978-3-642-71417-7 e-ISBN-13:978-3-642-71415-3
DOI: 10.1007/978-3-642-71415-3

Library of Congress Cataloging-in-Publication Data. Speech restoration via voice prostheses. Bibliography: p. . Includes index. 1. Artificial larynx. 2. Laryngectomees – Rehabilitation. I. Herrmann, I.F. (Ingo Ferdinand), 1942– . II. Amatsu, M. (Mutsuo), 1937– . RF538.S64 1986 617'.533 86-15610
ISBN-13:978-3-642-71417-7 (U.S.)

Softcover reprint of the hardcover 1st edition 1986

2122/3130-543210

List of Contributors

You will find the addresses at the beginning of the respective contribution

Preface

This book contains a series of articles and summaries regarding surgical voice restoration after or during a total laryngectomy. Most readers will recall the pleasure patients feel when they are able to speak again after years of mute existence.

A few simple questions are relevant to the articles contained herein. Firstly, how important is a person's voice? Is it for example as important to man as the dances bees use to convey essential information? Even the most superficial consideration must tell us that the function of the human voice is still more important as we already have a detailed body language of our own, e.g., when we feel pain, joy, love, fear, etc. Without doubt, speech is the basis of knowledge and surely it is the capacity to learn which characterizes the human intellect.

Secondly, one may ask whether man was always intended to have a voice? A few every-day observations can provide us with an answer. When little children play together, for instance, they all speak at once and seldom listen to what their neighbors are saying. Obviously, this is because it is not so important what they are actually saying as that something is being said at all.

Similarly, I recently overheard an elderly married couple chatting to each other. The man was talking about the weather but his wife answered by discussing one of her friends' problems. As he began to speak in greater detail about the weather, she replied that her sister was not taking her friend's problem seriously enough. Clearly, the deep need to speak simply for talking's sake does not depend on age.

Nearly everyone eventually says what is on their minds. We all talk about our experiences and few of us keep our thoughts entirely to ourselves.

A further question: Do we need a listener? I think we do or at least an imaginary one. It is a fact that we need to speak for a certain amount of time every day. Speech is a basic human instinct and a physiological necessity. After listening for any length of time it is almost impossible not to want to speak. One could almost compare such a compulsion with the need to eat and drink. The concept of speech as both a creative and life-giving activity was perceived as early as in Ancient Egypt. The Egyptians portrayed God the Creator as a chattering duck.

If voice restoration also enables a patient to satisfy a basic human need once again, the contributors to this book are engaged in more than mere technical reconstruction work. Indeed, they are promoting the very well-being and happiness of the patient. So 113 years after the first laryngectomy was performed, it is the worthy aim of this book to come a little nearer to answering some of the problems posed by voice restoration.

Furthermore, it is hoped that this book will encourage the reader and young doctors in particular, to find new ways to solve the centuryold problem of surgical voice rehabilitation.

Finally, I should like to thank all the various people who were involved in the production of this book and in particular the following: Mr. Guilleaume of the firm Xomed/Xomed Ltd. for his generous support; Mr. Dawson for his painstaking editing of the English texts; Mr. Bergstedt and team for the excellent arrangement of this book; and finally Mrs. Stark for her thorough compilation of the manuscripts.

I. F. HERRMANN

Contents

Chapter 5 Indications, Results and Their Means of Evaluation

Chapter 6 Speech Training, Intelligibility and Psychosocial Aspects

Chapter 7 Fingerless Voice Restoration

Historical Perspective

"Every cancer operation has been condemned on its first introduction and only after many failures does it find permanent surgical acceptance".

These words were spoken at the Society of Physics and Medicine in Würzburg on February 12th, 1882, by the surgeon Ernst von Bergmann in a lecture on laryngectomy. His positive view of the then new operational laryngectomy technique contradicted W. H. Horse in his monography "Is laryngectomy preferable to tracheostomy in cancer?" who condemned the operation as impracticable and irresponsible. Even in 1888, the Frenchman Demors censured that „La statistique de cette opération est une véritable martyrologie“ at the French Surgeons Congress in Paris.

This was the same year the German Kaiser Frederic the Third died after a, for the most part, conservative treatment of a laryngeal cancer by the Englishman Morell Mackenzie.

Nothing has changed to alter the basic facts of this "martyrdom" even today. A laryngectomy is still indicated when the extent of a tumor makes partial resection impossible or when it spreads from the hypopharynx into the larynx. The latter case is only recognized at an advanced stage because the tumors can grow for a long period of time in this part of the body without any accompanying symptoms. It is only when there is a fixation of the vocal folds and the patient begins to become hoarse that anything is noted.

In a laryngectomy, an 8 cm long segment is cut out which extends the air pipes cranially and connects the pharynx. This segment stretches from the hyoid bone to the first tracheal ring. The larynx has the following functions: respiration, phonation, aspiration protection, and – through the ventilation of the olfactory region – smell.

In December 1873, 15 years before the death of Kaiser Frederic the Third, Theodor Billroth carried out the first laryngectomy involving an extended laryngeal carcinoma. It was an emergency operation. The stencilled preparation shows clearly how the tumor had completey displaced the larynx. Billroth had to choose between performing a palliative tracheostomy to save the patient from asphyxiation or a radical tumor resection. He chose the latter and applied a large pharyngostoma i.e. he connected the pharyngeal mucous membrane with the outer skin. He then sutured the tracheal stump onto the outer skin. The patients who underwent this technique usually died prematurely of aspiration pneumonias as food, liquid, and saliva got into the air passages. In 1881, Gluck reported the successful separation of the pharynx from the trachea. He closed the pharynx and

Speech Restoration Via Voice Prostheses
Edited by I. F. Herrmann

left the tracheostoma. Patient prognosis improved dramatically. At last, air was blocked from the digestive tracts.

Simultaneously, Gluck also began to practise a voice rehabilitation technique with his patients which had already been created in France 40 years before the first laryngectomy. In 1856, Czerny referred to this technique in one of his publications. He meant, of course, the so-called oesophageal speech. Patients whose larynx had been displaced by acute stenosis or atresia and who had been provided with a tracheostoma learned to swallow air and to form words when it ascended. luck was therefore able to achieve a certain degree of voice rehabilitation.

Gussenbauer too, a pupil of Billroths, began to carry out voice rehabilitation after his first experiences with laryngectomy. He developed a special cannula with a chimney. This chimney was inserted in the pharyngostoma. Inhalation was affected via the cannula and exhalation via the chimney. A lid closed over the chimney during deglutition to avoid aspiration through the cannula. However, the seal of the pharyngostoma was not tight enough around the cannula and aspiration resulted.

Introduction

Over the last 100 years, many authors have attempted voice rehabilitation with a connecting canal between the respiratory tract and the digestive tract. Once the tracheostoma has been sealed, the air travels along the connecting canal and up into the digestive tract. The mucous membrane oscillates in the air stream at the point of transition between the open and the collapsed part of the pharynx to produce phonation. The exact position of the sound-producing segment depends on the type of technique used, e.g., on the extent of the resection. If only the larynx is resected, clip marks placed during the operation show that the sound-producing segment is on the same level as the upper edge of the thyreopharyngeal muscle. In the last few years, voice prostheses have been developed to avoid aspiration via the connecting canal between the respiratory tract and the digestive tract. They allow air to flow into the pharynx and prevent liquid getting into the trachea. E. D. Blom and M. I. Singer gave the fundamental impetus for the development of these new prostheses. It is the purpose of this book to present the various new prostheses and pass on the experience which has been gained with their usage (Chap. 1).

Experiments have shown that prostheses can be improved in quality by increasing their inner diameter and by altering their valve. Other parameters such as prosthesis length, valve position, prosthesis material, and position of the prosthesis opening on the side facing the respiratory tract are all of relatively minor importance for prosthesis resistance. However, the size of the inner diameter of the prosthesis is limited as higher prosthesis volume in the oesophagus impedes the digestive tract and makes shunt insufficiency possible by creating a disproportion between wall strength and prosthesis diameter. Fungi, bacteria, and food particles cover and develop into the silicon of the prosthesis. Any research which deals with the above problems will help towards a better understanding of the function and handling of voice prostheses and their complications. A. Schauer gives a detailed account of prosthesis material compatibility in the article found later in this book (Chap. 2).

Once the prosthesis is in place, the necessary phonatory resistance is composed of two elements. Experiments have therefore been conducted to measure prosthesis resistance and pharyngeal resistance. Pharyngeal resistance can be calculated by subtracting the known prosthesis resistance from the total resistance found in vivo. Research results have been presented in this book to further illustrate the interrelationship between the prosthesis and the pharynx (Chap. 3).

In some patients, a strong hypertrophy of the inferior pharyngeal constrictor muscle has been observed either immediately or several months after the insertion

Speech Restoration Via Voice Prostheses
Edited by I. F. Herrmann

of the voice prosthesis. This impeded phonation to a considerable extent and patients could only speak with high pressures. Attempts were made by myotomies, muscle denervation viz. muscle elimination or by two of these methods to solve this problem. So-called functional pharyngeal surgery was thus developed to maintain voice modulation, i.e., oesophageal contractility. Extensive efforts to deal with this constriction problem have shown that successful and reliable patient rehabilitation cannot be guaranteed by prosthesis insertion alone. J. Lang describes the relevant functional anatomy in his later contribution. The various solutions proposed to solve this problem need to be confirmed by other researchers (Chap. 4).

Surgical voice rehabilitation techniques presented so far must be critically compared with the extensive field studies available for voice rehabilitation with oesophageal speech. Snidecore reports in his comprehensive monograph, in which he compiles all the relevant world literature, that between 43% and 68% of patients attain sufficient voice rehabilitation with oesophageal speech after laryngectomy. Over 300 patients have been supplied with various different types of valve prosthesis at the Universities of Groningen and Würzburg. 88% of these patients have satisfactory phonation. The results reflect a quantitative improvement. Various proposals have been made to measure voice quality. Questions have been raised as to the possibility of establishing a generally-accepted procedure to measure the voice quality of the surgical voice rehabilitation obtained by different research groups and techniques (Chap. 5).

One fundamental problem is discussed in the chapter on the psychosocial aspects of voice rehabilitation. Comparisons between the different rehabilitation capacities found in patients help researcher better to understand the quantity and quality of their results. The patients' own remarks are most instructive (Chap. 6).

Ways have also been sought to achieve fingerless phonation. New values and operating techniques have enabled the first steps to be made towards fingerless phonation with the aid of tracheostoma valves. The possibility of rehabilitation without foreign bodies, surgery, or finger occlusion have also been discussed. The results obtained so far to be confirmed (Chap. 7).

One important finding in the psycho-social studies is the considerable limitation experienced by the patient with a permanent tracheostoma. In 1969, Kluyskens was the first to try to solve the problems of a permanent tracheostoma viz. loss of smell by trying to perform a larynx transplant. The transplant required immuno-suppressive treatment which unfortunately stimulated renewed tumor growth. The result of these experiments was a world-wide debate as to the justification of such surgical procedures. It was decided at the time that larynx transplants with immuno-suppressive treatment had to be abandoned. As the larynx is not a vital organ, the risk of a transplant is considered disproportionally high. Since then no further experiments have been made to tackle this serious tracheostoma problem which greatly hinders the patient in his work and social life. In a series of initial trials, attempts have been made to insert a changeable artificial larynx in animals. Preliminary results are to be presented soon (Chap. 8).

Chapter 1 The Different Types of Voice Prostheses

The Simple Semi-Permanent Supratracheal Valve Prosthesis after Total Laryngectomy

E. MOZOLEWSKI, K. JACH, C. TARNOWSKA and A. DALEK [1]

The first report of an internal valve prosthesis was published by our department in 1972. We presented a general outline of our method and results.

Our endoprosthesis is handmade for each individual patient. It takes the form of a tube made either from stiff polyethylene or from a more elastic polyvinyl. Its internal diameter is 3–5 mm (Fig. 1). The inner end of the tube has a simple external pressure valve. It is 3–5 mm long and consists of 2–3 layers of polyethylene foil 0.007 mm thick. The foil is welded onto the polyethylene tube and pressed onto the polyvinyl one by the polyethylene flange. This flange prevents both prosthesis dislocation and leakage around the tube. A similar one is fastened to the outer end of the prosthesis after its introduction into the tissue. The introduction procedure of the prosthesis is shown in Fig. 2.

The shape of the prosthesis depends on the anatomical or pathophysiological conditions in any particular case. Usually, a short 1.3–2.0 cm long tube was used with the internal outlet under the pharyngoesophageal sphincter (Fig. 3). In the case of high sphincter pressure, the inner end of the prosthesis was directed upwards and place close to the sphincter's upper border.

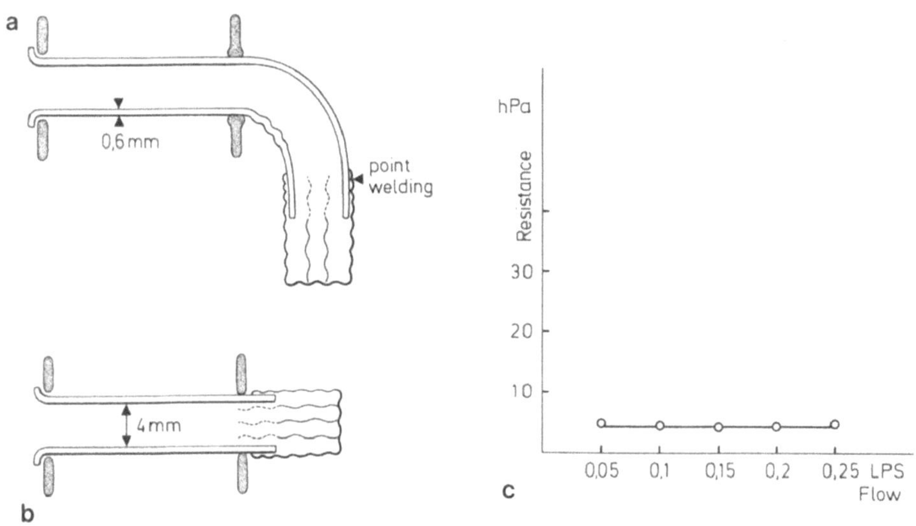

Fig. 1. Cross-section of the prosthesis and its airflow resistance in vitro

[1] Ul.Unii Lubelskiej Nr. 1, 71–344 Szczecin, Poland.

Speech Restoration Via Voice Prostheses
Edited by I. F. Herrmann

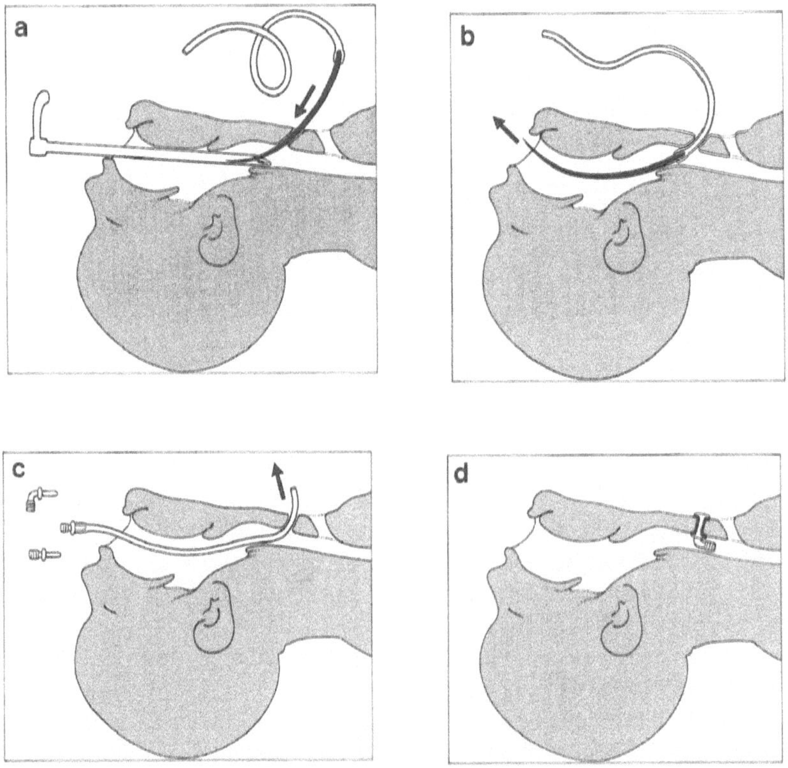

Fig. 2. Insertion of the prosthesis: **a** introduction of the oeseophagoscope and perforation of the soft tissue just above tracheostoma with a long needle connected to a polyvinyl drain (O.D = 5 mm); **b** movement of the needle and drain through the pharynx and mouth; **c** mounting of prosthesis on the drain and pulling it downwards; **d** prosthesis in correct position

Our prosthesis can last for years. Only when the valve had to be directed upwards did we have to charge it after several months. To charge the prosthesis, we first cut away the external security flange and mount the rest of the prosthesis on the elastic catheter. We then push the catheter and prosthesis through the mouth. The new prosthesis is fastened to the catheter and correctly introduced into position through the mouth. The whole procedure does not burden the patient but requires a trained physician.

In contrast to the intratracheal puncture usually performed today, we prefer to work through the skin just above the tracheostomy. We can thus avoid massive penetration of tracheobronchial secretion into the prosthesis. This is important because the prosthesis material does not possess any self-cleaning properties. None the less, some crusting at and around the external outlet of the prosthesis means that the patient must clean it daily. Irrigation is seldom necessary.

Depending on the state of the tracheostoma region, expiratory air can be directed into the prosthesis for phonation either by thumb pressure or by a concave screen. This screen is about 3 cm in diameter and is either worn freely about the neck or permanently connected to a tracheostomic tube.

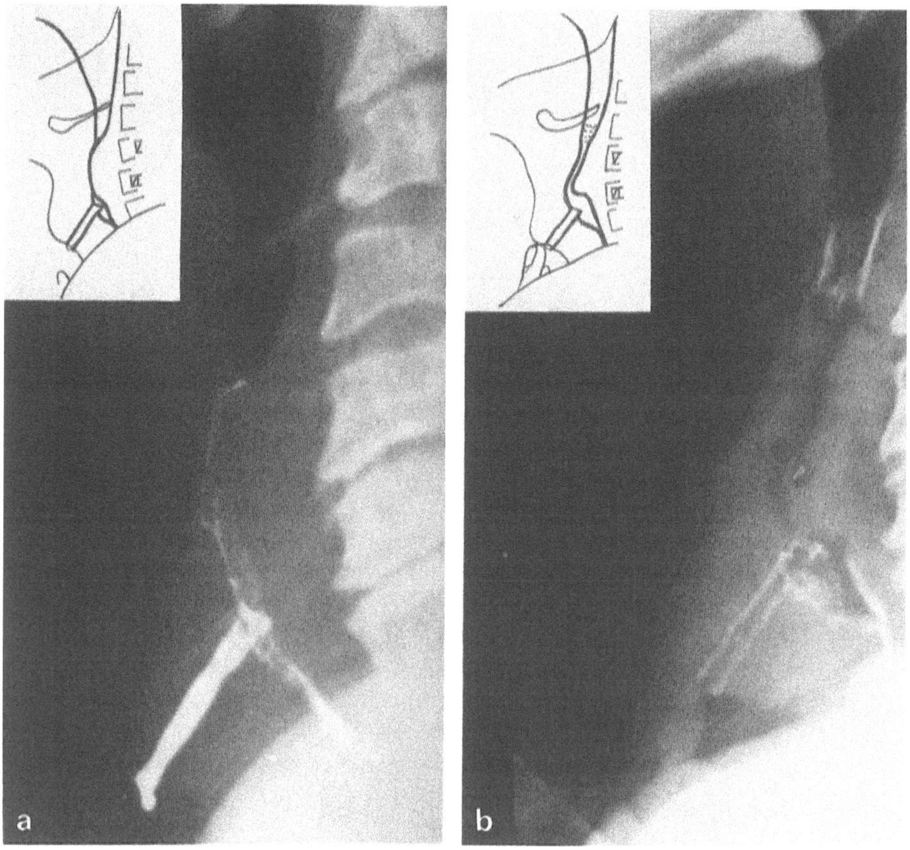

Fig. 3. X-ray of the pharynx with the prosthesis at rest and during phonation

This prosthesis was only used as a secondary procedure in 26 cases. Its local biocompatibility was found to be good in all cases. After 6 months the opening around the tube started to broaden and liquids and saliva began to leak in one patient with a thin cervical wall. After removal of the tube, the shunt closed without any other necessary procedure. In the second case after typical formation of the shunt, the canal was about 3 cm long at the pathway and strongly flexed. 7 months later an abscess of the neck was formed which completely drained away after the prosthesis was removed. Apart from unwanted local reactions the prosthesis had to be removed for one patient as an early local neoplasm reoccurred. Another patient removed the prosthesis local neoplasm reoccurred. Another patient removed the prosthesis himself because he thought it was making him hiccup. Up till then, the patient had good oesophageal voice. Our longest observation period is 12 years without any change of prosthesis. After several years, a ring of moderate hyperthropic fibrous tissue was observed around the prosthesis.

During normal conversation 10 patiens used an expiratory air pressure of $\bar{x}=$ 36,0 kPa (25–50 kPa), flow $\bar{x}=0$, 127 Lps (0,05–0,25 Lps) with a loudness of (at a distance of 1 m) $\bar{x}=71{,}8$ dB (60–82 dB). A softer voice was observed at lower

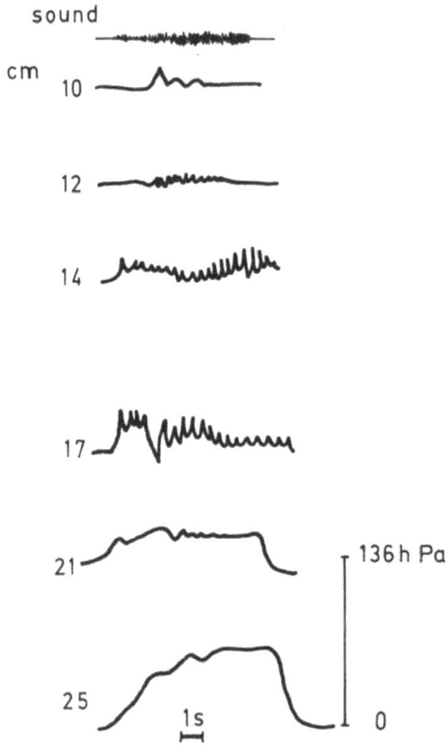

Fig. 4. Perfusion manometry of the pharynx and oesophagus during phonation. Patient G. B. 8 months after a total laryngectomy with primary myotomy and 3 weeks after a secondary insertion of the prosthesis. Resting pressure absent. During phonation: high pressure increase in the middle part of oesophagus (25 cm from incisor teeth) due to wall contracture. Lower increase in the upper part of the oesophagus (21 cm) due to filling up with expiratory air. Slight increase in pressure combined with vibrations in the area of the myotomized pharyngo-oesophageal sphincter (14–17 cm) disappearing in the upper parts of mesopharynx

pressure following the myotomy of the pharyngo-oesophageal sphincter. The resistance of the whole system, taking prosthesis resistance in vitro into account should be mainly related to the source connected with the pharyngo-oesophageal high pressure zone. In our manometric investigations of the pharynx and oesophagus after laryngectomy, it was found that the anterior-posterior resting pressure in that zone amounts to 90:136 KPa. Following a myotomy with an interposition of the thyroid gland, the pressure at rest was strongly reduced whereas it was increased during phonation. The acoustic phenomena were connected with vibrations observed at the outlet of the elevated pressure zone (Fig. 4).

The perceptual and acoustic characteristics of speech were measured by phoniatric examination and spectrographic analysis. Phoniatric examination was carried out on all 26 patients and spectrographic analysis in only 9 cases. In all cases, the voice was perceived to be low-pitched and slightly hoarse.

After an adjustment period of several weeks voice could be produced freely and with some melodic elements. The average phonation of the vowel "a" was 13 s (8.15 s). The average intelligibility during the word tests was 84%. Scores ranged from 58%–98%. The number of syllables was 240–270 per min. The spectrographic analysis of 9 cases distinguished two types of excitation: (a) periodic-aperiodic excitation approximating to normal phonation in 3 cases, and (b) periodic-aperiodic excitation with a predominant nasal component in 6 cases. Noise intensity did not influence segmentation. The average basic frequency was 95 Hz. The individual average F_0 ranged from 80 to 100 Hz. The basic frequency ranged during word utterance from 25 to 55 Hz ($\bar{x} = 34$ Hz). On the musical scale the average range of basic frequency included tones (min. 3, max. 9). In all cases, the lowest formants F_1 and F_2 were 200–300 Hz higher than the normal voice.

Discussion

Our hand-made valve prosthesis after laryngectomy has proved useful for 15 years. However, we use it seldom in our patients as we employ oesophageal voice or autoplastic vocal shunts wherever possible. The advantages of our type of valve prosthesis are its durability, very low airflow resistance, anatomical adaptability and readily available low-cost material. This last feature may prove to be important in countries where the cost of the often more convenient but less durable industrially produced prosthesis is prohibitive.

The disadvantages of our prosthesis are: (a) Its poor self-cleaning ability of tracheo-bronchial secretion which makes it necessary to introduce this device through the skin above tracheostoma. This position still causes some problems regarding the deflection of the expiratory air stream into the prosthesis. (b) The great stiffness of the flanges which complicate prosthesis change. (c) The time taken for its construction and fitting in individual patients.

Summary

To summarize, we are convinced that the industrially produced prosthesis with its self-cleaning properties, high elasticity, and high biocompatibility is more convenient that our own prosthesis. However, useful practical results can be obtained with our prosthesis which sometimes exceed those of other prostheses (Weinberg 1982; Zietek et al. 1978).

The perceptual and acoustic characteristics of speech obtained with our valved prosthesis resemble those found after autoplastic shunts with the internal orifice below or in the pharyngo-oesophageal sphincter (Tarnowska 1980). Its quality is still not as good as the speech obtained by an autoplastic shunt with the internal orifice in the pharynx (Tarnowska et al. 1982). The quality of speech produced with our prosthesis was far better than that produced by the classic oesophageal one. After a surgical procedure on the pharyngo-oesophageal sphincter or myotomy with interposition of the thyroid gland (Mozolewski et al. 1984), there was usually no such difference. The most striking difference between the two kinds of speech was in the time it took to train the patients. Those with a prosthesis start to speak immediately after insertion, whereas the mastering of oesophageal speech usually requires at least several weeks of intensive training and a strong motivation on behalf of the patient (Tarnowska et al. 1982) even after a primary plastic procedure on the sphincter. Good oesophageal speakers believe that they are better off than the patient provided with a prosthesis despite slightly worse speech fluency. We believe that the difference in speech quality is too small to justify the effort of caring for the prosthesis. Probably, professional speakers would not share this opinion. At present the most important problem to be solved with the low pressure prosthesis is the great amount of energy needed for phonation due to the poor transformation of air stream input energy into acoustic output energy of a desirable quality. We believe that real progress might be made with a better control of the morphology and action of the pharyngo-oesophageal high pressure zone. We were able to prove this for oesophageal speech (Mozolewski et al. 1984; Tarnowska et al. 1982).

Our supratracheal semi-permanent valve prosthesis has been used since 1969. Its aerodynamic properties in vitro and in vivo as well as its tissue compatibility are reported. Particular attention is paid to phonation problems regarding energy consumption as well as perceptual and acoustic voice characteristics.

References

Barton RT (1965) A review of attempted physiological restoration of voice following total laryngectomy. Proc. VIII Int. Congr. ORL Tokyo

Blom ED et al. (1982) Tracheostoma valve for postlaryngectomy voice rehabilitation. Ann Otol Rhinol Laryngol 91:576

Conley JJ (1970) Concepts in head and neck surgery. Thieme, Stuttgart

Edwards N (1975) Post-laryngectomy vocal rehabilitation using expired air and an external fistula method. Laryngoscope 85:690

Herrmann IF (1982) personal communication

Jach K (1979) Physical parameters of vocal shunt phonation in laryngoctomized. Polish. Ann Acad Med Stet 25:492

Lebrun Y (1967) Über den künstlichen Kehlkopf. Z Laryngol Rhinol Otol 46:389

Mozolewski E (1972) Surgical rehabilitation of voice and speech after laryngectomy. Polish. Otolaryng Pol 26:654

Mozolewski E et al. (1972) Studies on formation of pseudoglottis after surgical rehabilitation of voice and speech. Otolaryngol Pol 26:663

Mozolewski E et al. (1984) Myotomy with interposition: its technique and results. Polish. Otolaryng Pol

Nijdam HF et al. (1982) A new prosthesis for voice rehabilitation after laryngectomy. Arch Otorhinolaryngol 237:27

Panje WR (1981) Prosthetic vocal rehabilitation following laryngectomy = the voice button. Ann Otol Rhinol Laryngol 90:116

Shedd D et al. (1972) Reed fistula method of speech rehabilitation after laryngectomy. Am J Surg 124:510

Singer MI, Blom ED (1980) An endoscopic technique for restoration of voice after laryngectomy. Ann Otol Rhinol Laryngol 89:529

Tarnowska C (1980) Phoniatric evaluation of shunt phonation. Ann Acad Med Stet 26:455

Tarnowska C et al. (1982) An attempt of comparison of alaryngeal speech after classical and surgical methods of rehabilitation. Otolaryng Pol 36:215

Tarnowska C et al. (1984) Esophageal voice following myotomy of pharyngo-esophageal sphincter. Otolaryng Pol

Taub S, Bergner LH (1973) Air bypass voice prosthesis for vocal rehabilitation of laryngectomees. Am J Surg 125:748

Weinberg B (1982) Airway resistance of the voice button. Arch Otolaryngol 108:498

Weinberg B et al. (1982) Airway resistance during esophageal phonation. J Speech Hear Disord 47:194

Zietek E et al. (1978) Intubated vocal shunt. Ann Acad Med Stet Suppl 15, 24, 35

A Second Generation Artificial Larynx Prosthesis – A Comparative Clinical Evaluation

J. N. HAUSFELD [1] and J. L. HENLEY-COHN [2]

The clinical feasibility of a controlled tracheoesophageal fistula for generation of fluent esophageal speech was first pioneered by the work of Drs. Singer and Blom. We have however encountered many practical difficulties with the use of voice prostheses. Problems encountered include extrusion, speech initiation delay, leakage around the prosthesis, stoma obstruction, and low volume output.

A second generation laryngeal prosthesis is introduced for comparison. Its design incorporates features that will significantly improve the clinical problems encountered; extrusion is minimized; the new prosthesis allows for one size to fit all patients; and the prosthesis remains in place for several months at a time.

A clinical trial was established to directly compare the artificial speech generated by the currently existing laryngeal prosthesis. Each laryngectomy patient was fitted with three different devices and the resulting speech was evaluated. Video recordings of patients are presented to illustrate the type of speech produced by each device. Comparisons of intelligibility, fluency, volume, and patient preference are made. Results indicate that a significant variation in speech obtained is critically dependent on the choice of prosthesis.

Introduction

A technique based on the insertion of a purged valve into a controlled tracheoesophageal fistula has been popularized over the past several years by Drs. Singer and Blom. The merit of this technique is its simplicity and lower complication rate. The technique is applicable to patients who have undergone total laryngectomy many years ago and who, because of persistent lack of appropriate communicative skills, require additional rehabilitation. In analyzing the result of many clinical studies, it always appears that the results achieved seem to be better in the hands of the physicians who contributed to the development of the primary device rather than in the hands of secondary investigators. This most likely reflects the fact that experience and confidence with a particular prosthesis, patient selection, and trained support services produce better results. The purpose of this study was to see which of the three currently available esophageal puncture devices in the United States produce the best speech reliably and have the least complications regarding its use. The three devices differ in their silicone makeup and style as well as the differences in the preferred positioning of each device.

[1] 1145-19th Street, N.W., Washington DC 20036, USA.
[2] New Haven, Connecticut 06510, USA.

Speech Restoration Via Voice Prostheses
Edited by I. F. Herrmann

Some of the clinical problems universally encountered include: leakage around the tracheoesophageal fistula, difficulty in initiating speech, stoma obstruction, crusting, difficulty in maintenance and care of the device. There appears to be a definitive patient population who, in spite of a successful and well-fitted device, still have difficulties in initiation of speech related to spasm of the middle constrictor musculature. The middle constrictor spasm in some patients plays an important role in prevention of fluent tracheoesophageal speech irrespective of the device used. It is because of this that all patients who were included in this study were asked to try to produce speech without any device in place and with a patent tracheoesophageal fistula. Many times it was found that the difficulty in speech initiation was device related and in these instances the second generation laryngeal prosthesis was helpful in obtaining fluent speech. In select patients, pharyngeal myotomy is an essential adjunctive procedure in the rehabilitation of the aphonic laryngectomy patient.

It has been our goal to resolve some of the difficulties encountered with the currently available laryngeal devices. A study involving laryngectomy patients fitted with the three different devices was established; clinical acceptance, patient compliance, speech fluency, and intelligibility were compared.

Device Development

Mathematical modelling techniques were used in the design of valve tip to help minimize opening pressure and maximize air flow. A mainframe Computer Aided Design (CAD) unit was used in the design of the device injection mold. A mold injected silicone device was constructed as illustrated in Fig. 1. The device has key features that help resolve some of the clinical difficulties encountered.

The inner flange functions as a retainer. The valve tip was designed specifically to minimize opening pressure and maximize air-flow, yet retain the integrity of

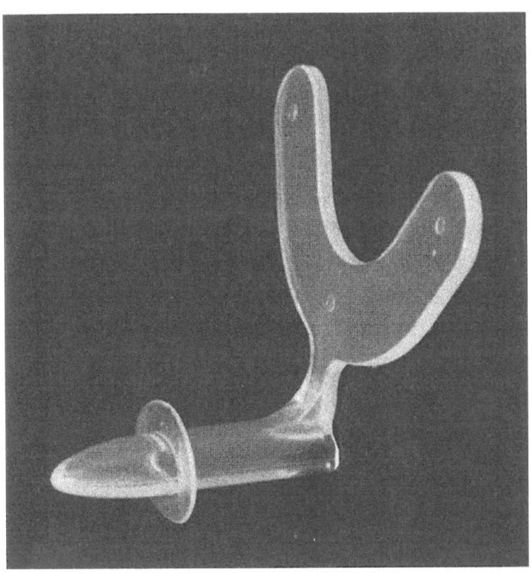

Fig. 1. Mold injected device made from HTR Silastic

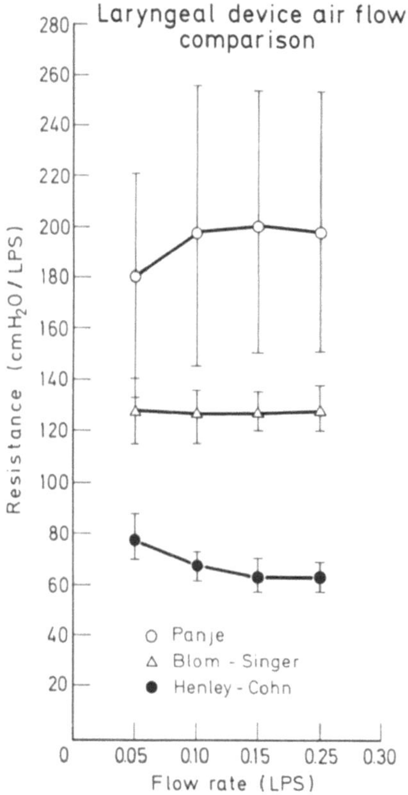

Fig. 2. Resistance versus flow graphs as measured in a laboratory. (Reproduction by permission from Robert Hillman et al., Boston University Medical School)

a one-way configuration (Fig. 2). The valve tip is self-cleaning and highly resistant to corrosion by saliva or absorption of lipids so often encountered and requires frequent cleaning in other devices. To be more specific, the low opening pressure, as well as resistance to lipid absorption and corrosion, is a Dow Corning proprietary developing of the silicone material that has been successfully used in hydrocephalus shunt valves. The outer flanges are larger than the tracheostomy to prevent inadvertent aspiration. They are placed medially to the SCM muscle clavicular insertions to prevent the extrusive force that is associated with neck rotation or flexion. One size device will fit all the patients, if the tracheoesophageal fistula is placed within 3 mm of the superior mucocutaneous stoma margin. These design features have allowed us to place the device in all encountered patients without fitting difficulties (Fig. 3).

These devices do not require daily removal. Cleaning is done by the patient, with the device in place. The HTR doped silicon has successfully retained its valve integrity for up to 8 months at a time, without removal of the device during the day or night. Because of the variability from patient to patient, we still recommend that a new device should be inserted at 3–4 month intervals. Additional work is being done with special silicone compounds to prolong this period even longer. Table 1 summarizes some of the relative advantages and disadvantages of each device.

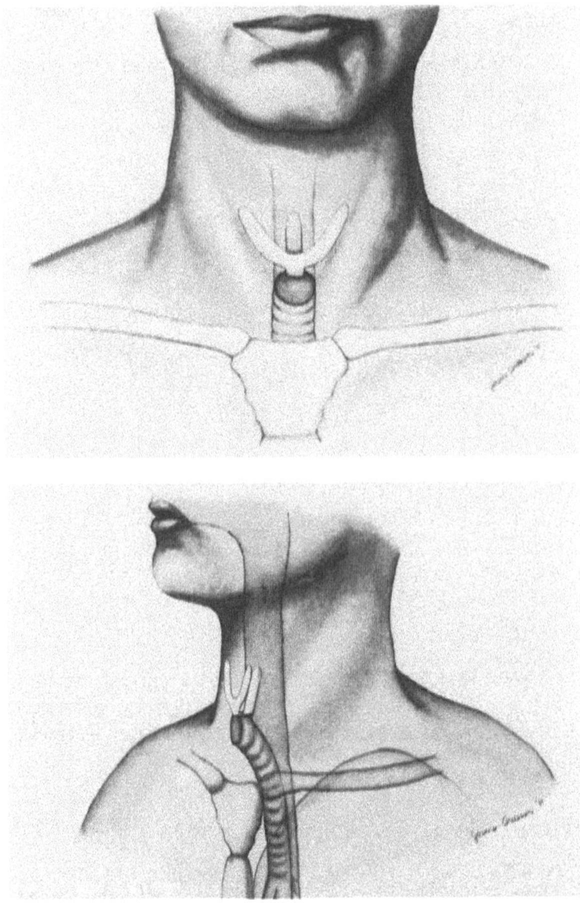

Fig. 3. Preferred positioning of device. Note the absence of stoma obstruction

Table 1. Tracheoesophageal laryngeal device comparison

Characteristic	Bivona Singer-Bloom	Xomed Panje	Dow Corning H-C
Opening pressure	Low	High	Very low
Air flow	Medium	Low	High
Extrusion rate	High	Low	Low
Stoma obstruction	Yes	No	No
Valve crusting	High	High	Low
Self care difficulty	Moderate	Moderate	Minimal
Post-op visits	Many	Many	Few
Patient training	Moderate	Moderate	Minimal
Speech fluency	Good	Fair	Very good
Speech volume	Good	Fair	Very good
Speech strain	Some	Moderate	Minimal
Device removal	Daily	Daily	2–3 months

Comparing available laryngeal devices, it becomes clear that the Singer-Blom device has a relatively low opening pressure but requires careful fitting. There are many different sizes available and extensive experience is necessary to achieve appropriate fitting. There are specific techniques involved in taping in a wet field around the tracheostoma which is critical to proper function of the device. A recently introduced inner flange may improve some of these problems. The device suffers from extrusion with neck flexion or rotation and patients with small tracheostomas may have crusting and air-way difficulties. The Panje button suffers from high opening pressure and difficulty in speech initiation. The valve is susceptible to lipid absorption as well as crystallization corrosion requiring removal and frequent cleaning.

Methods

A comparative study was established with seventeen laryngectomy patients that had already been fitted with either a Singer-Blom prosthesis or a Panje Button. Each of these patients had some difficulty with the currently existing device which usually resulted in speech production. However, sometimes problems with stoma obstruction and valve crusting were encountered. Initially, the existing device was removed and the patient was asked to attempt to phonate through the patent tracheoesophageal fistula without any device in place. This was done to assess whether or not the problem in speech generation was device related or secondary to spasm of the constrictor muscles. Then the patient was fitted with the other devices and was given ample time to practice with these devices after which time a video recorded interview was utilized to assess the nature of the speech generated. A comparative reading was made on each patient testing all three devices. A patient was first tested with a Singer-Blom-device (properly fitted) in place then switched over to a Panje Button, and then switched to a HC device. With a small population of patients it is hard to quantify this and the video recordings are submitted for demonstration. Obviously this kind of preliminary study would have to be verified by other investigators. These studies are currently in progress.

Discussion

In our clinical experience with existing devices over the past several years, it has become apparent that strong support from experienced speech pathologists was essential for success when using the Singer-Blom or Panje prosthesis. A device that remains in place, does not extrude or obstruct and performs flawlessly for at least 3–4 months would be of great advantage to a clinician without such support. A speech pathologist can then concentrate on patient speech therapy instead of daily maintenance, cleaning, taping and adjustments of the laryngeal device. The design parameters discussed above have clearly established that both speech fluency and patient compliance are markedly improved with the second generation prosthesis. All patients were given a choice of which device to use on a daily basis. Greater than 80% of those tested preferred the H-C device (12 H-C device, 2 Singer-Blom device, 1 Panje device, and 2 no device at all).

Investigators concentrating on the design and function of future devices should not overlook a critical factor in the rehabilitation of these patients played by the middle constrictor musculature. It has been our clinical experience that for a number of patients who are unable to generate any significant speech, a pharyngeal constrictor myotomy – either performed at the time of the laryngectomy or as a separate procedure – produced vast improvements. As an illustration, a video recording is made of the patient (who is completely unable to speak) with the device in place. Temporary speech was achieved with a Xylocaine blockade of the middle and inferior constrictor musculature and lasted for about 15 minutes. This patient underwent middle constrictor myotomy and his rehabilitated speech was fluent and highly intelligible.

Conclusion

A comparative study of seventeen laryngectomy patients with three different tracheoesophageal devices was performed. These patients were initially having difficulty in generating good speech with the Singer-Blom or Panje devices and many of these patients were able to become highly intelligible with the use of a second generation H-C device. Video recordings were utilized to assess the nature, volume, intelligibility and fluency of speech. The design parameters of this laryngeal prosthesis were discussed in detail.

Surgeons who are not successful in rehabilitating their patient after a tracheoesophageal puncture should first determine whether or not the problem is related to the device selected or to spasm of the constrictor musculature. This is done by having the patient attempt to phonate with no device in place and assess the nature of speech generated. If there is a great degree of spasm of the constrictor musculature then no device which is available will be able to overcome this obstacle. A constrictor myotomy performed on these patients will result in a greater percentage of laryngectomized patients who will be able to achieve fluent esophageal speech. If it is felt that the problem is device related either in regards to the opening pressure of a certain device or to its positioning in the stoma or the patients ability to maintain daily care, then the surgeon should opt to try different devices which are currently available.

As you can see from the other papers in this publication, there is rapid progress being made in this field. This study points out the evolution from the initial devices to the newly emerging prosthesis which are now available. Just as the surgeon has many stapedectomy prostheses to choose from, he will now be able to select from a variety of different tracheoesophageal devices. Each of these may have its own particular advantages or disadvantages for a selected patient but in all will add to our armamentarium in obtaining fluent speech in the laryngectomized patient.

References

Donegan JO et al. (1981) Limitations of the Blom-Singer technique for voice restoration. Ann Otol Rhinol Laryngol 90:495–497
Gates GA et al. (1982) Current status of laryngectome rehabilitation. I. Results of therapy. Am J Otolaryngol 3:1–7
Henley-Cohn J (1981) How I do it: Head and neck: New technique for insertion of laryngeal prosthesis. Laryngoscope 91:1957–1959
Komisar A, Hoch L (1982) Rehabilitation of speech following tracheoesophageal puncture. Laryngoscope 92:1126–1129
Maran AJ et al. (1982) Management techniques in the use of the Blom-Singer valve. Clin Otolaryngol 7:201–211
Maves MD, Lingerman RE (1982) Primary vocal rehabilitation using the Blom-Singer and Panje voice prosthesis. Ann Otol Laryngol 91:458–460
Panje WR et al. (1981) Voice button prosthesis rehabilitation of the laryngectomee. Additional notes. Ann Otol Rhinol Laryngol 90:503–505
Perry A et al. (1982) A modification of the Blom-Singer valve for restoration of voice after laryngectomy. J Laryngol Otol 96:1005–1011
Shapiro MJ, Ramanathon VR (1982) Tracheostoma vent voice prosthesis. Laryngoscope 92:1126–1129
Singer MI et al. (1981) Further experience with voice restoration after total laryngectomy. Ann Otol Rhinol Laryngol 90:498–502
Weinberg B (1982) Airway resistance of the voice button. Arch Otolaryngol 108:498–500

The Groningen Voice Prosthesis for Secondary Voice Rehabilitation after Total Laryngectomy

H. F. NIJDAM[1], A. A. ANNYAS[2], H. K. SCHUTTE[2] and H. F. MAHIEU[2]

The problem of an open tracheo-oesophageal fistula which would allow air to pass in one direction without aspiration remained unsolved until Singer and Blom (1979) developed a technique using a valved silicon prosthesis. A similar biflanged silicon prosthesis was introduced later by Panje (1981).

These devices have several advantages over purely surgical techniques: Simplicity, minimal morbidity, and a high rate of successful speech rehabilitation. The main disadvantages of these prostheses are the stenting of the newly created tracheo-oesophageal fistula several days prior to prosthesis insertion, the daily removal and reinsertion of the prosthesis for cleaning purposes, the danger of accidental dislodgement, and the need to use adhesives for fixation of the prosthesis.

The Groningen voice prosthesis was therefore developed in 1980. The prosthesis shape resembles a biflanged tube. The tracheal side is made like a flange with a small string (Fig. 1). The string is only used to insert the prosthesis and is removed later. The tracheal side of the prosthesis is open. The oesophageal side resembles a combined flange and one-way valve. The large valve outlet was developed to allow the passage of sufficient quantities of air from the trachea to the oesophagus and to stimulate self-cleaning properties in the prosthesis. The passage of air during speech production removes all secretion from the inside of the shaft and valve.

The one-way valve can pivot slightly on the shaft and enables good adaptation to the proximal part of the oesophagus. The shaft length is available in 7 sizes (3, 5, 7, 8, 9, 11, and 13 mm) and allows an exact fit with each type of fistula.

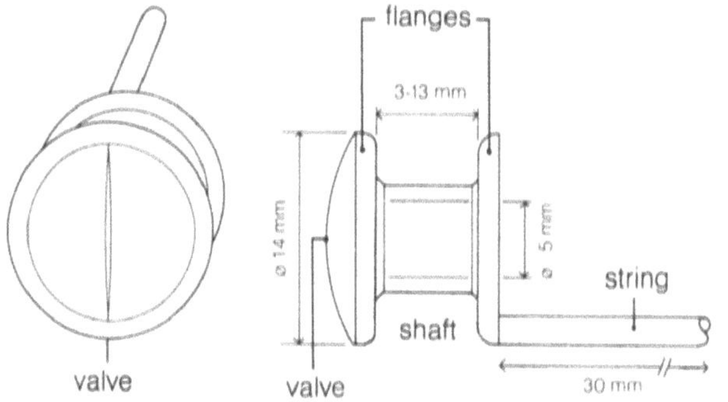

Fig. 1. The Groningen voice prosthesis. Shaft length comes in 7 sizes: 5–13 mm

[1] Juliana v. Stolberglaan 4, 1623 ME Hoorn, The Netherlands.
[2] Academic Hospital Groningen, 9700 RB Groningen, The Netherlands.

Speech Restoration Via Voice Prostheses
Edited by I. F. Herrmann

Because of the dimensions of the valve on the oesophageal side, the voice prosthesis has to be inserted via the mouth and the oesophagus. Some instruments were developed especially for this procedure, i.e., a grasping forceps with a blunt or sharp tip and a puncturing trocar. Nowadays, the puncturing trocar is seldom used; tracheo-oesophageal puncture is performed with the sharp grasping forceps.

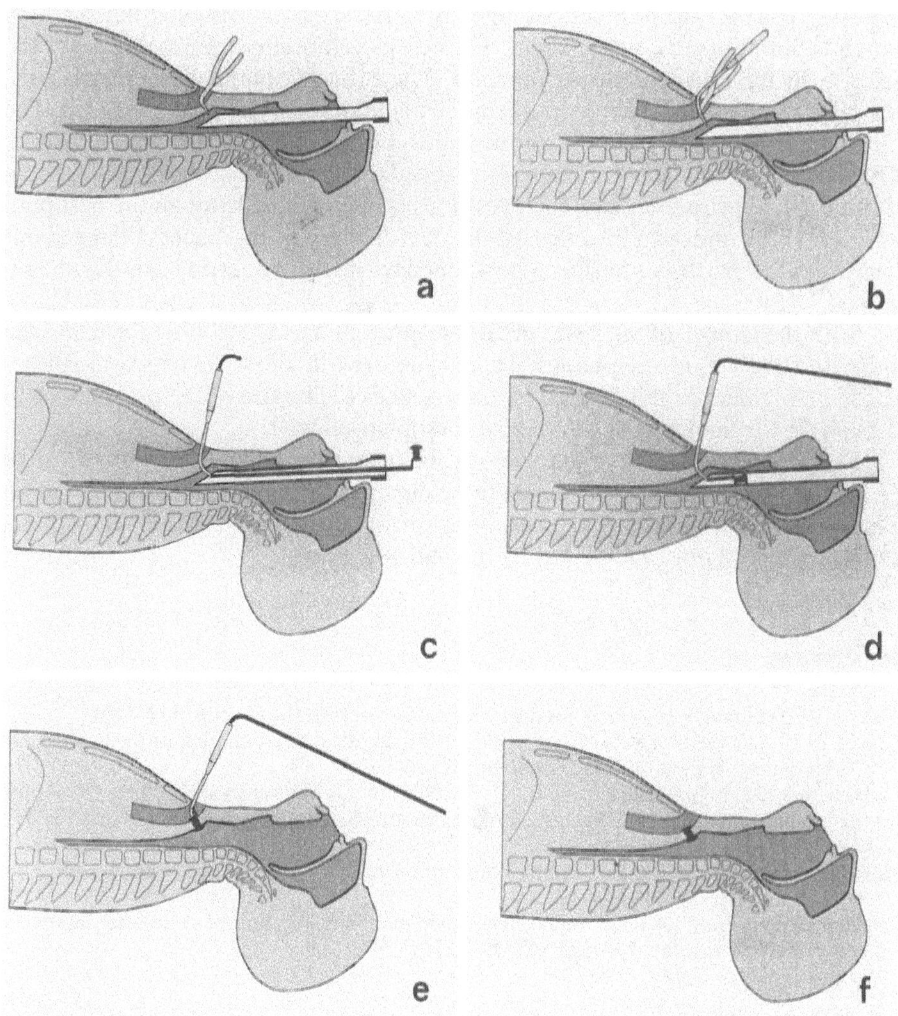

Fig. 2. **a** Perforation of the tracho-oesophageal wall into the oesophagoscope. **b** Introduction of the flexible grasping forceps through the fistula. **c** Attachment of the voice prosthesis string to the grasping forceps. **d** The voice button is withdrawn into the oesophagoscope. **e** Insertion of the prosthesis into the fistula. **f** After insertion, the silicon string is removed

Methods

Oesophagoscopy is carried out under local or general anaesthesia. The oesophagoscope is placed 2 cm below the tracheostome (Fig. 2). Transillumination through the tracheo-oesophageal wall as well as palpation of the tip of the oesophagoscope are useful for orientation purposes. The oesophagoscope is rotated 180° in order to bring the bevelled surface directly behind the posterior tracheal wall. The fistula is then created by making a puncture through the posterior tracheal wall into the oesophagoscope, using the specially designed sharp grasping forceps or the puncturing trocar. The best puncture site is approximately 1 cm inferior to the mucocutaneous junction. The rotated oesophagoscope prevents the posterior oesophageal mucosa from being injured by the puncturing tip. The flexible grasping forceps are introduced into the oesophagoscope via the fistula. The sharp tip of the flexible forceps is attached to the silicon string of a voice prosthesis of an appropriate size. The prosthesis is then passed through the oesophagoscope and withdrawn into the fistula. The delivery of the tracheal flange confirms that the prosthesis has been positioned correctly. The string can then be removed.

Both the flanges of the voice prosthesis prevent accidental dislodgement into either the trachea or oesophagus. There is no need to allow the fistula to epithelialize beforehand as it is stented by the prosthesis. The size of the prosthesis will depend on the thickness of the tracheo-oesophageal wall.

The prosthesis functions on average for over 3 months within a total range of 1–21 months. The prosthesis has to be changed at the end of its working life. This is easily done under local anaesthesia on an out-patient basis. The prosthesis cannot and need not be removed by the patient.

References

Asai R (1972) Laryngoplasty after total laryngectomy. Arch Otolaryngol 95:114–119

Conley JS et al. (1958) A new surgical technique for the vocal rehabilitation of the laryngectomized patient. Ann Otol Rhinol Laryngol 67:655

Gussenbauer C (1874) Über die erste durch Th. Billroth am Menschen ausgeführte Kehlkopf-Exstirpation und die Anwendung eines künstlichen Kehlkopfes. Arch Klin Chir 17:343–356

Panje WR (1981) Prosthetic vocal rehabilitation following laryngectomy – the voice button. Ann Otol Rhinol Laryngol 90:116–120

Singer MI, Blom ED (1980) An endoscopic technique for restoration of voice after laryngectomy. Ann Otol Rhinol Laryngol 89:529–533

The Groningen Voice Prosthesis for Voice Rehabilitation During Total Laryngectomy

H. F. Nijdam [1], A. A. Annyas [2], K. T. van der Laan [2] and H. K. Schutte [2]

Speech loss is the most distressing side-effect of total laryngectomy. Voice rehabilitation through learning oesophageal speech by injection is still the most preferred method for speech restoration after total laryngectomy as this does not increase the length of the operation.

However, a certain percentage of patients are unable to learn this phonation method. Therefore, such patients welcome surgical or prosthetic voice restoration techniques. The most widely-advocated surgical technique today is the Staffieri and Serafini (1976) technique which involves the creation of a tracheo-oesophageal fistula lined with oesophageal mucosa. The main problems connected with this neoglottic shunt are leakage of saliva or food and spontaneous closure of the fistula (Leipzig 1980). The most widely-used prosthetic techniques (Singer and Blom 1980; Panje 1981) recommend that the fistula is stented for several days prior to prosthesis insertion.

The Groningen voice prosthesis (Nijdam et al. 1982) was primarily developed for use during total laryngectomy. The tracheal flange and a combined one-way valve and flange on the oesophageal side mean that the prosthesis itself is used as a stent in the tracheo-oesophageal fistula. The various shaft lengths (2, 5, 7, 8, 9, 11, and 13 mm) enable an exact adaptation to the thickness of the tracheo-oesophageal wall.

Method

The operative technique required to insert the prosthesis during total laryngectomy does not differ essentially from the one described for secondary techniques (Nijdam et al. 1982). The same sharp grasping forceps are employed.

A normal or wide field total laryngectomy is performed. Pre-operative radiotherapy or unilateral and bilateral neck dissection are carried out where necessary. At the end of the operation while the hypopharynx is still open, the tracheostoma is made by suturing the trachea into the skin. The tracheo-oesophageal puncture is then performed and preferably with sharp grasping forceps. The puncture is directed towards a finger in the proximal part of the oesophagus. The sharp grasping forceps are advanced through the fistula into the hypopharynx. In the open wound, the voice prosthesis is connected to the tip of the grasping

---

[1] Juliana v. Stolberglaan 4, 1623 ME Hoorn, The Netherlands.
[2] Academic Hospital Groningen, 9700 RB Groningen, The Netherlands.

Speech Restoration Via Voice Prostheses
Edited by I. F. Herrmann

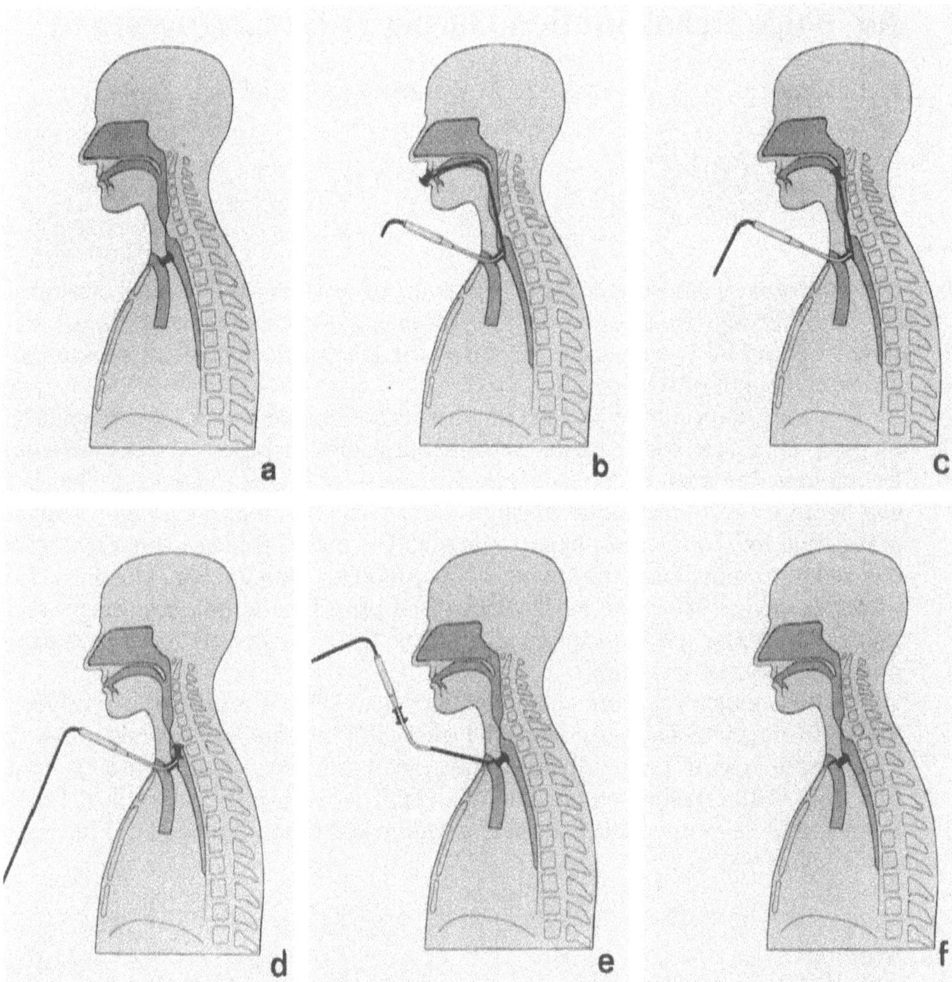

Fig. 1. Changing of the voice prosthesis at the end of device life: **a, b** Introduction of the blunt flexible grasping forceps under local anaesthesia. **c, d** The new voice prosthesis being drawn into the oesophagus. **e, f** Dislodgement and removal of the old voice prosthesis and insertion of the new one

forceps and drawn into the fistula. The string on the prosthesis is removed when correctly positioned. The procedure adds approximately 5 min to the operation.

When extensive parts of the hypopharyngeal mucosa have to be removed during operation or the proximal part of the oesophagus is constricted, it is advisable to perform a crico-pharyngeal myotomy. While keeping the finger in the oesophagus, the muscle fibres of the constrictor muscle are cut down to the mucosa and as far caudal as possible. The operation is then finished in the normal way.

After 10–12 days, the gastric tube is removed and the patient is allowed to speak via the fistula. Successful speech production then depends not only on anatomical factors but also on the mental condition of the patient. When the patient is carefully instructed beforehand as to what kind of speech and feelings he can expect to have after the operation, he will realy always learn to speak. Speech therapy is advisable to achieve maximum voice results in each patient.

At the end of prosthesis device life (commonly indicated by mild leakage through the prosthesis and concomitant coughing), a new voice prosthesis has to be inserted (Fig. 1). This can be done under local anaesthesia on an out-patient basis. The pharynx and trachea are sprayed with an anaesthetic solution. Then the blunt grasping forceps are introduced into the oesophagus through the old voice prosthesis and advanced into the mouth. The tip of the forceps is attached to the string of the new prosthesis and drawn into the oesophagus. The old prosthesis is then dislodged using a curved hemostat, and the new prosthesis inserted in the fistula. This procedure ensures that the new prosthesis is correctly positioned with its one-way valve in the oesophagus and its tracheal flange in the trachea.

References

Leipzig B (1980) Neoglottic reconstruction following total laryngectomy. A reappraisal. Ann Otol 89:534–537

Nijdam HF et al. (1982) A new prosthesis for voice rehabilitation after laryngectomy. Arch Otorhinolaryngol 237:27–33

Panje WR (1981) Prosthetic vocal rehabilitation following laryngectomy – the voice button. Ann Otol 90:116–120

Singer MI, Blom ED (1980) An endoscopic technique for restoration of voice after laryngectomy. Ann Otol 89:529–533

Staffieri M, Serafini I (1976) La riabilitazione chirurgica della voce e della respirazione dopo laryngectomia totale. 29th National Congress of the Associazione Otologi. Ospedalieri Italiana Bologna. Associazione Otologi Ospedaliere Italiana, pp 57–111

The Groningen Button Results

H. F. Mahieu [1], A. A. Annyas[1] and H. F Nijdam [2]

Introduction

In 1980, the first Groningen button was placed in a patient undergoing a total laryngectomy in the ENT-department of the Groningen University Hospital.

The two main reasons for developing this new device, which enabled tracheo-oesophageal fistula speech production, were firstly that no other device was commercially available in Europe at that time, and secondly that a device was needed which would stay in place for a longer period of time without having to be removed by the patient for daily cleaning purposes. By contrast, the need to develop a device for tracheo-oesophageal fistula speech production seemed less urgent as our speech rehabilitation programme already achieved a very high standard of conventional oesophageal speech, with 85% of the patients developing good or moderate injection oesophageal speech (determined using the criteria proposed by Schutte et al. 1984). This is an excellent result compared with other studies (Gates et al. 1982; Schaeffer and Johns 1982). However, the first speech rehabilitation results with the Groningen button proved to be far superior to those with the conventional injection oesophageal speech method. Therefore we soon decided to place a Groningen button in the majority of patients undergoing a total laryngectomy. Only patients with extremely poor manual dexterity and unlikely to achieve sufficient stoma occlusion, or patients with severe chronic obstructive pulmonary disease were not considered for button method speech. The Groningen button was placed as a secondary procedure using the endoscopic technique in a small number of patients who had already been laryngectomized before the Groningen button was available and who had been unable to achieve satisfactory injection oesophageal speech. The value of a non-laryngeal speech device can be measured by the number of patients who attain good speech ability. However, if one wants to evaluate the quality of such a device or to make a qualitative comparison between various different devices, the complications and the patient's reactions should also be taken into account. Several aspects regarding the speech quality of patients using the Groningen button are discussed in another paper (Mahieu et al. 1985). Therefore, only the subjective evaluation of speech quality is dealt with in this paper.

[1] Academic Hospital Groningen, 9700 RB Groningen, The Netherlands.
[2] Juliana v. Stolberglaan 4, 1632 ME Hoorn, The Netherlands.

Speech Restoration Via Voice Prostheses
Edited by I. F. Herrmann

Results

83 patients received the Groningen button at the ENT-department of the Groningen University Hospital either during or after a total laryngectomy from December 1980 to June 1984. Patients with a follow-up period of less than 3 months were excluded from this study. Patients who were unable to follow our speech rehabilitation program due to early tumor recurrence or postoperative complications, which were not due to the Groningen button, were also excluded from this study. This left us with 71 patients who were available for evaluation. This group of patients consists of 66 males and 5 females with a mean age of almost 61 years at the time of the total laryngectomy. The follow-up period varies from 3 months to 3.5 years, during which period no essential changes were made in the silicon plastic material of the Groningen button. All the patients except one received preoperative radiotherapy with an overall dose of 30 Gy, and 19 patients received an additional postoperative dose of 30 to 40 Gy. The speech rehabilitation programme begins as soon as possible which generally means the 10th postoperative day when the naso-gastric feeding tube is removed in the case of a patient who received the Groningen button during total laryngectomy and the first postoperative day if the button was placed later with an endoscopic technique. All patients began training with both the conventional injection method and the button method of speech simultaneously. 54 patients received the Groningen button during total laryngectomy. In 17 patients, the Groningen button was placed at a later date which varied from several weeks to 10 years after total laryngectomy. The Groningen button was removed from 38% of the patients, i.e., 19 patients who underwent a primary procedure and 8 patients who received the button later. The main reason for a patient's request to have his button removed was the smaller use of the button-assited oesophageal speech when they had mastered good injection oesophageal speech. It is interesting to note that almost all patients who had their button removed claim that the button method of speech was louder, more fluent, and more intelligible than the injection method of speech. They also report that the Groningen button was very useful for them especially in the beginning. More than 70% of the patients were able to speak with the button method immediately during the first day of the speech rehabilitation programme. This compares with 10% of patients with the injection method. Furthermore, the button method proved to be less influenced by emotional stress than the injection method of speech. The louder more fluent speech of the button method with less stoma noise is especially favourable in the beginning when the injection speech method has still not yet been fully mastered. When comparing the results of the injection and button method of speech, we asked trained speech therapists to evaluate patients' speech as "good", "moderate" or "poor". It is important to note that the criteria used for the button method are much stricter than the criteria used for the injection method of speech. In other words, a "good" or "moderate" score for button method results indicates a much better voice than a "good" score for the injection method of speech. The reasons for the differences between the strictness of these criteria are discussed in a paper by Schutte et al. (1984). Of these patients, 55 were rated as having "good", 7 "moderate" and 9 "poor" speech with the button method. This same group had 27 "good", 16 "moderate", and 28

"poor" speakers with the injection method of speech. The good and moderate speakers with the button method represent 87% of the total patient group, a success rate which is comparable with other published results. On the other hand, only 61% of these patients achieved good or moderate speech ability with the injection speech method.

Recently, all patients, including those from whom the button had already been removed, were asked if they were, or had been satisfied with the Groningen button. There is a significant difference between the number of satisfied patients who received the button from 1980 to 1982 and those who received the button during the last two years. 35% of the patients in the former period were not satisfied, which is a rather poor result. This compares with only 5% in the latter period which is a very good result. The majority of the dissatisfied patients can be divided into 2 groups:

1. Those patients who received the Groningen button more than 1 year after total laryngectomy. Often the quality of both the injection method and the button method of speech was poor in this group. For the 17 patients who received the Groningen button after total laryngectomy, a negative correlation exists between the number of satisfied patients and the period of time which elapsed from the laryngectomy to the actual placement of the button. The longer the period, the less patients are satisfied with the result. Of the seven patients who had the button placed more than 2 years after the laryngectomy, only one patient was satisfied with the result.
2. The second group of dissatisfied patients consists of those who had a persisting fistula after removal of the button. Most of these patients were not dissatisfied at the time of the button removal, but developed problems at a later date. Of the 27 patients who had their button removed, only 13 had a tracheo-oesophageal fistula which closed spontaneously within 10 days after removal. One fistula closed spontaneously after 4 weeks, and the remaining 13 patients had to undergo a surgical fistula-closing procedure. The longer the Groningen button had been situated, the smaller the number of fistulas which tended to close spontaneously. The normal surgical fistula-closing procedure with fistula excision and twin-layer suturing was often not successful. Therefore, a technique was developed using the interposition of a dermal graft as described by Annyas and Escajadillo (1984). All 8 of the dermal graft fistula-closing procedures performed were successful.

The main reasons for the difference between the number of satisfied patients from 1980 to 1982 and those of the last 2 years are that since 1982 Groningen buttons have no longer been placed more than 1.5 years after total laryngectomy and that since 1983 the dermal-graft method for closing of the fistula has been used if the fistula does not close spontaneously within 10 days. Furthermore, it is obvious that the patients benefit from the accumulating experience of the medical team. This is a further explanation for the difference in the number of satisfied patients.

As far as the device itself is concerned, our experience shows that the mean lifetime of the Groningen button is more than 3 months. During this period, the device does not have to be removed for cleaning purposes etc. Groningen buttons that stay in place for longer periods are not exceptional. So far the longest period has been 22 months. Figure 1a shows a patient with a Groningen button which

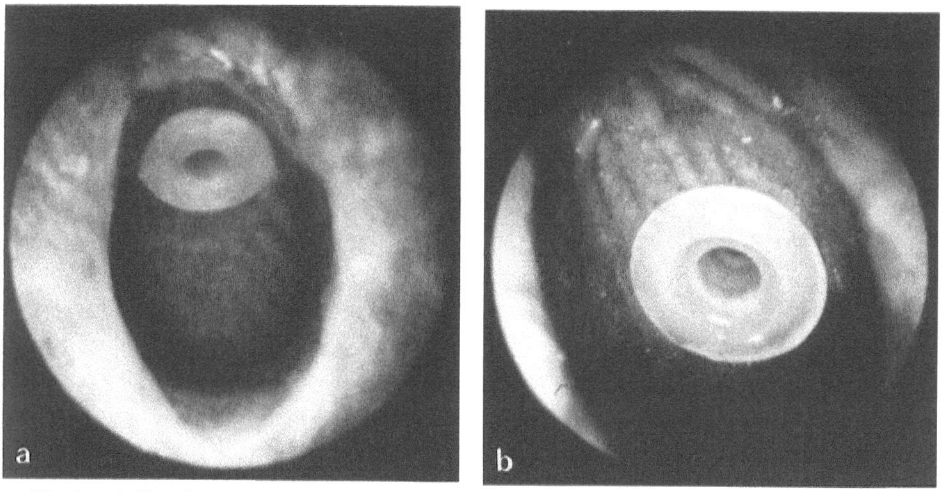

Fig. 1. a A Groningen button 12 months in situ. **b** Idem 19 months in situ

has been in place for over a year. Figure 1 b shows another patient with a button which has been in place for 19 months. The end of the device life is indicated by mild leakage through the valve part of the button or by increasing airflow resistance of the valve part forcing the patient to produce higher expiratory air pressures when using button-assisted oesophageal speech. The expiratory air pressure required can be measured in the tracheostoma and values of up to 20 kilopascal on loud phonation are sometimes found. These expiratory air pressures are subject to large individual variation. Most patients complain of headaches and poor button-assisted oesophageal speech production when airflow resistance is too high towards the end of the device life. The major cause of this increasing airflow resistance and mild leakage seems to be some sort of deposit found on the oesophageal flange (which is also the valve part) of the button. Why some patients acquire more button deposits than others is still unknown. However, we have been able to determine that these deposits are not lime-deposits and that they do not adhere to the surface of the silicon plastic material but have actually interacted with the material itself. This suggests that these "deposits" are actually chemical combinations of the silicon plastic material.

Complications

Complications with the placement to the Groningen button were not found during total laryngectomy or endoscopic procedure. Complications with the Groningen button were also not observed in the immediate postoperative period. Changing the Groningen button has also not given rise to complications. Buttons were changed more than 450 times due to mild leakage or increasing airflow resistance. 10 changes had to be made under general anaesthesia, but not in the last 2 years. Once a new puncture had to be made because a stenosis of the fistula had

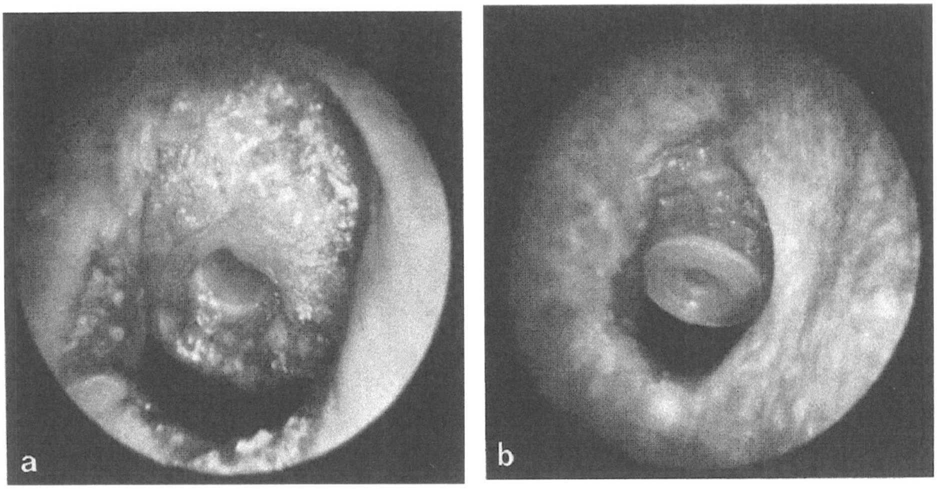

Fig. 2. a Hypertrophic mucosa in trachea. The Groningen prosthesis is nearly visible. **b** Same patient 14 days after replacement with a longer button

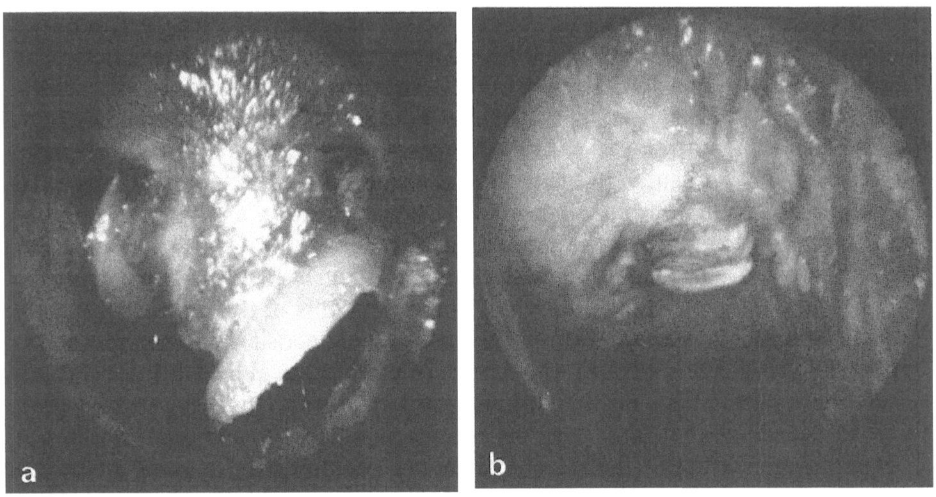

Fig. 3. a Hypertrophy and infection of the mucosa with dislocation of the button towards the trachea. **b** Same patient 1 week after removal of the button. The tracheo-oesophageal fistula has closed

occurred after the patient had lost his button without knowing it. In 15 cases, patients mostly lost their button by swallowing, but there were no cases of button aspiration. 6 patients complained of intermittent leakage from between the fistula wall and the Groningen button. As this was due to a widening of the tracheo-oesophageal fistula, the leakage was successfully treated in two ways. Either a button with a larger tube part diameter was used, or the button was temporarily removed from the fistula until the fistula shrank again, which always occured within 3 days. Hypertrophic tracheal mucosa was seen in about a quarter of the patients. This never bothered the patients and spontaneous regression usually occurred when a longer button was introduced. Figure 2a shows a patient with a mass of hypertrophic tissue, which almost obscures the Groningen button. The patient made no complaints. Figure 2b shows the same patient two weeks after the placement of a longer button. In one patient, the hypertrophic tissue had to be removed surgically. This was complicated by local infection which displaced the button towards the trachea as can be seen in Fig. 3a. This was the only patient where the button had to be removed due to local infection. Figure 3b shows the situation 1 week after the patient had also been treated with antibiotics. The fistula closed spontaneously. As this patient no longer used the button method of speech, no new puncture was performed. In four other patients, a mild local infection occurred which reacted favorable to antibiotic treatment. Two patients developed a candida albicans infection of the oesophagus. Both cases were successfully treated with ketoconazol.

Discussion

Although the placement of the Groningen button resulted in a high percentage (86%) of functional speech communication ability, a large number of patients (38%) wanted to have the button removed after a certain period of time. Almost all of these patients had acquired good injection oesophageal speech as well as good button-assisted oesophageal speech. Despite the fact that the button method of speech was louder, more fluent, and more easily intelligible than the injection method of speech, these patients preferred to use injection-oesophageal speech, because no stoma occlusion with either a finger or tracheostoma valve is necessary. A considerable number of patients gradually preferred the injection method of speech more and button-assisted oesophageal speech less. This was to be expected bearing in mind the high standard of injection oesophageal speech achieved in our clinic. Sometimes these patients were not even aware of this gradual change in their speech method preference. An impaired self-cleaning function of the Groningen button results because this can only work when air passes through the device regularly. If the button is not used regularly, i.e., at least several times a day, airflow resistance will increase. This not only causes the patient discomfort when speaking with the button method but also impairs his speech quality. Both of these effects contribute to the patient's preference for the injection method of speech. It is remarkable that almost all of the patients were still satisfied with the results of the Groningen button at the time of the button-removal. They were glad that the button had been placed during total laryngectomy as the ability to speak almost immediately after the operation proved to be a great encouragement to further speech rehabilitation and resocialization. More than 70% of the patients were dismissed from hospital only two weeks after total laryngectomy with the button method of speech. Such rapid speech rehabilitation does not generally occur with the injection method. Many patients were able to learn the injection method of speech in a more relaxed manner because they were already able to express themselves with the button speech method. The number of patients in this study who achieved good or moderate speech quality with the injection method (61%) seems rather small compared to the percentage of patients (85%) with the good or moderate injection speech production found in our speech rehabilitation programme over the last ten years. There are two reasons for this discrepancy. First of all, a negative selection was made as 17 patients, who are included in the study, received the Groningen button after total laryngectomy. This secondary procedure was performed because these patients had poor injection oesophageal speech production. Secondly, some patients who had already attained good voice production with the button method were less motivated to learn the injection method of speech because the latter method is harder and takes longer to learn.

Conclusions

Patients profit the most from the Groningen button if it is placed during total laryngectomy. It is a reliable device with few complications and enables good speech production. Only 5% of the patients who have received the Groningen button in the last two years were unsatisfied; nevertheless, it is advisable to teach patients both the injection method and the button method of speech because a considerable number of patients decide to use the injection method once they have fully mastered it, which is usually after about a year.

Contraindications for the placement of the Groningen button are:

- extremely poor manual dexterity with doubtful stoma occlusion;
- severe chronic obstructive pulmonary disease producing large amounts of pulmonary secretions and causing crusting around the device;
- when a period of more than 1.5 years has lapsed since total laryngectomy. This tentative conclusion is based on the fact that most patients in this study who received the button after this period were not satisfied with the results.

References

Annyas AA, Escajadillo JR (1984) Closure of tracheoesophageal fistulas after removal of the voice prosthesis. Laryngoscope 94:1244–1245

Gates et al. (1982) Current status of laryngectomee rehabilitation. 1. Results of therapy. Am J Otolaryng 3:1–7

Mahieu HF et al. (1984) Intelligibility, vocal intensity and LTAS of the Groningen button oesophageal speech. In: Speech restoration via voice prosthesis. Int Workshop June 1984, Würzburg

Schaeffer SD, Johns DF (1982) Attaining functional oesophageal speech. Arch Otolaryng 108:647–649

Schutte HK et al. (1984) Evaluation of speech with and without a "Groningen type" voice button. In: Speech restoration via voice prosthesis. Int Workshop June 1984, Würzburg

Voice Rehabilitation after Laryngectomy with the Groningen Voice Prosthesis: Experiences Made in Nijmegen

J. J. MANNI, P. VAN DEN BROEK and M. A. H. DE GROOT [1]

Introduction

Shortly after Blom and Singer (1979) and Singer et al. (1981) began to discuss the results of a simple tracheo-oesophageal puncture technique with the combined insertion of a valved prosthesis, we began using this method in our department. The Blom-Singer prosthesis was only used in 9 patients, however, as the Groningen voice prosthesis was developed soon afterwards, we decided to adopt the Groningen voice prosthesis (Nijdam et al. 1981) because it was more simple than the other prosthetic device techniques available in 1981 and because it could be inserted during laryngectomy. The purpose of this paper is to report on the experiences we have made with this prosthesis towards vocal rehabilitation after total laryngectomy.

Methods and Patients

The Groningen voice prosthesis is described in detail by Dr. Nijdam. The prosthesis can be placed in the tracheo-oesophageal wall during laryngectomy, as a primary operation, or a secondary procedure some time after surgery (Nijdam et al. 1982).

The precise surgical procedure is outlined in this book. To summarize, the insertion of the Groningen voice prosthesis is a onestage procedure needing no secondary interventions. The prosthesis is self-retaining, self-cleaning, and remains in situ for an average of 3 months. It can be changed in the out-patients department. Between November 1981 and February 1984, 34 patients underwent primary and 6 patients secondary vocal rehabilitation with the Groningen voice prosthesis after total laryngectomy.

In the primary group (mean age 63), 16 patients received a short course of intensive preoperative radiation (25 Gy in 5 days; Kazem et al. 1982). 4 of these patients underwent a postoperative radiation therapy of up to 65 Gy with the prosthesis in situ. The other patients all had tumors which recurred after a full course of radiotherapy. 12 of these 34 patients underwent a unilateral and 2 a bilateral neck dissection in conjunction with the laryngectomy. In the group undergoing secondary voice rehabilitation (mean age 54), 2 patients received 25 Gy preoperative radiation treatment and 4 were radiation treatment failures.

[1] St. Radboudziekenhuis, 6500 HB Nijmegen, The Netherlands.

Speech Restoration Via Voice Prostheses
Edited by I. F. Herrmann

In our opinion, primary prosthetic rehabilitation might be indicated in all cases of laryngeal carcinoma where there has been total laryngectomy. This method was contraindicated for subglottic tumor extension, postcricoid carcinoma, massive postradiation oedema and suspected radiation perichondritis. It was also contraindicated for pulmonary emphysema, chronic bronchitis, and manual impairment. The secondary procedure could be performed when oesophageal speech is poor or unintelligible. Further contraindications are too large tracheostoma and excessive coughing against the stomal capping. Other contraindications were career or hobbyrelated ones, e.g., where the patient was a farmer, gardener, or cook. Speech therapy was usually begun within 3 weeks of a primary and 1 week of a secondary procedure.

Results

The insertion of the Groningen voice prosthesis as a primary procedure prolonged the laryngectomy by less than five minutes. The secondary procedure performed under general anaesthesia, lasted an average of 8 min. All patients were able to be discharged from hospital the day after the operation without needing a feeding tube, special diet or antibiotics.

Intelligible, versatile and fluent speech with a reasonable dynamic vocal range was used as a basis to evaluate rehabilitation success. Patients were independently evaluated by a speech therapist, an ENT-surgeon, and a medical student.

In 2 of the 34 patients, the prosthesis had to be removed within the minimum post-insertion observation period of 3 months. Removal was indicated because of severe coughing in one case and permanent fear of stomal capping in another. Successful speech rehabilitation was achieved in 26 of the 32 remaining patients. The prosthesis was removed after varying periods in all 6 of the failures. 5 now use an electrolarynx and one has achieved a moderately intelligible oesophageal speech. In the group with secondary rehabilitation, successful speech was achieved in only 3 of the 6 patients.

In Table 1 technical proficiency data for the first 10 patients rehabilitated with the Groningen voice prosthesis are compared with the oesophageal speech results of various Dutch laryngectomees reported by van den Berg et al. (1958).

Table 1. Comparison between the technical proficiencies of sound production by oesophageal speech (van den Berg et al. 1958) and Groningen voice prosthesis (the authors)

	Oesophageal speech	Groningen prosthesis
Maximum loudness	50–70 dB	74–102 dB
Dynamic range	20 dB	6– 28 dB (mean 22 dB)
Phonation duration	3– 8 s (mean 3 s)	3– 31 s (mean 10.5 s)
Syllables per injection	3– 5	12– 30 (105)[a]

[a] Excluded.

Fig. 1. Replacement of the Groningen voice prosthesis; a simple outpatient procedure under local anaesthesia: **a** Introduction of flexible metal device through the shaft of the old prosthesis towards the oral cavity; **b** the new prosthesis is attached extraorally to the metal device; **c** removal of the old prosthesis, unusual surface deposits; **d** insertion of new prosthesis. **e** The string is out and the new prosthesis is drawn in situ; **f** the flange is cut

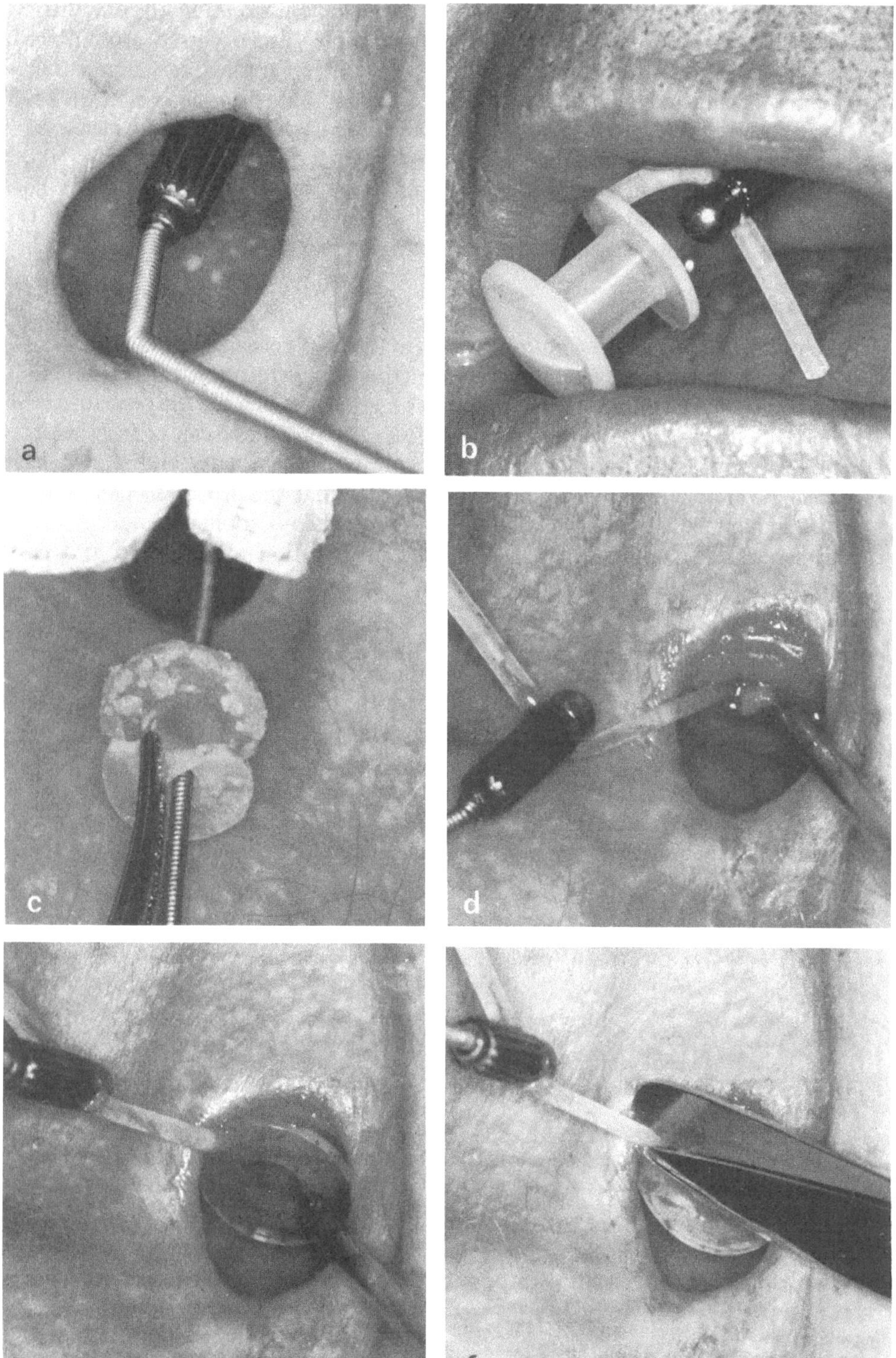
a
b
c
d
e
f

No aspiration of food or liquid was observed. On one occasion, the prosthesis was dislodged by excessive coughing. Granulations also occurred around the prosthesis but were treated successfully. Prosthesis replacement is a simple outpatient procedure which can be performed under local anaesthesia and only takes a few minutes (Fig. 1). Replacement is indicated for any leakage of fluid, increased transprosthesis air pressure resistance, or speech deterioration. In our study, the prosthesis remained in situ for an average of 4 months (range: 1–9 months). The fistula site usually healed of its own accord within 4 days of permanent removal. In 6 occasions, however, surgical closure was necessary.

Discussion

Recently-developed devices for insertion into the tracheo-oesophageal wall seem to be improvements on current operative methods to restore voice after total laryngectomy. The Groningen voice prosthesis has been used since 1981 because we believed it superior to other available devices. The prosthesis can be inserted as a primary procedure during total laryngectomy. Both primary and secondary placement are one-stage procedures. This means that the prosthesis can be inserted simultaneously with the puncture of the tracheo-oesophageal wall. As the prosthesis is self-retaining and self-cleaning, daily insertion is unnecessary and patient instruction is minimal. However, the patient cannot replace the prosthesis himself.

In this study, 26 of the 32 patients could speak after a primary procedure compared with 3 out of 6 patients after a secondary procedure. The negative selection of the secondary group may be responsible for the poor results. Radical neck dissection or previous radiation did not influence the results. The results correspond to previous reports by both Hilgers et al. (1983) and Annyas et al. (1984). In conclusion, voice rehabilitation with the Groningen voice prosthesis should be considered a good alternative method to prosthetic speech rehabilitation. No complications were encountered which could be attributed to the insertion or use of this prosthetic device.

Acknowledgment. Mr. J. Meeuwissen (Dept. of Medical Illustrations at the University of Nijmegen) provided the photographs.

References

Annyas AA, Nijdam HF, Escajadillo JR, Mahieu HF, Leever H (1984) Groningen prosthesis for voice rehabilitation after laryngectomy. Clin Otolaryngol 9:51–55

Berg JW van den, Moolenaar-Bijl AJ, Damsté PH (1958) Oesophageal speech. Folia Phoniat (Basel) 10:65–84

Blom ED, Singer MJ (1979) Surgical prosthetic approaches for postlaryngectomy rehabilitation. In: Keith RL (ed) Laryngectomee rehabilitation. College Hill Press, Houston

Hilgers FJM, Schouwenburg PF, Scholtens B (1983) Herstel van de spraak na totale larynxextirpatie; chirurgische en prothetische mogelijkheden. Ned Tijdschr Geneeskd 127:1120

Kazem J, Broek P van den, Huygen PLM (1982) Planned preoperative radiation therapy for advanced laryngeal carcinoma. Int J Radiation Oncology Biol Phys 8:1533–1537

Nijdam HF, Annyas AA, Schutte HK, Leever H (1982) A new prosthesis for voice rehabilitation after laryngectomy. Arch Oto-Rhino-Laryngol 237:27–33

Singer MJ, Blom ED, Hamaker RC (1981) Further experiences with voice restoration after total laryngectomy. Ann Otol Rhinol Laryngol 90:498–502

Staffieri M, Procaccini A, Steiner W, Staffieri A (1978) Chirurgische Rehabilitation der Stimme nach Laryngectomie. Laryng Rhinol 57:477–488

The Phoniatric Results of Our Voice Prostheses (36 Cases)

L. TRAISSAC, M. LECOQ, J. PETIT, F. DEVARS, I. IGNATOV, J. Y. NIZOU, M. BENKIRANE and F. MOUROT [1]

Our voice prosthesis was used in 36 patients when there were the following indications:

- Failure of Staffieri's neoglottis in 12 cases:
  8 because the neoglottis was too wide,
  4 because the neoglottis was too narrow (voice was difficult or impossible).
- Failure of Staffieri's shunt (tracheo-oesophagus) a long time after total laryngectomy in 8 cases:
  2 because the shunt was too wide
  4 because of stenosis
  1 because of a prior unsatisfactory prosthesis insertion
  1 because of placement a long time after failure of the shunt (stenosis)
- Placement during total laryngectomy in 13 cases.
- Placement a long time after total laryngectomy and unsuccessful oesophagus voice training in 3 cases.

Prosthesis and Placement Techniques

1. The Prosthesis

All prostheses used in these 36 cases were manufactured by ourselves in the operation room with deep-feeding tubes. This is therefore an experimental study. This experience enabled us to advance in prosthesis manufacture and to find more convenient and reliable prostheses.

a) Our prosthesis is divided into two parts (Fig. 1): The higher pharyngeal part and the lower tracheal part. These two parts are adjusted by sliding one into the other and allow us to adapt the length of the tube to each patient as far as possible.
b) Each of the two parts has a collarette at each end which enables good stability and avoids aspiration.
c) There is also a valve on the pharyngeal side to avoid aspiration but its suppleness allows air flow for phonation.
d) The higher pharyngeal part extends in the form of a tube which acts as a guide on its way through the tracheo-oesophageal wall after placement.

[1] 89 Rue des Sablières, F-33077 Bordeaux Cedex.

Speech Restoration Via Voice Prostheses
Edited by I. F. Herrmann

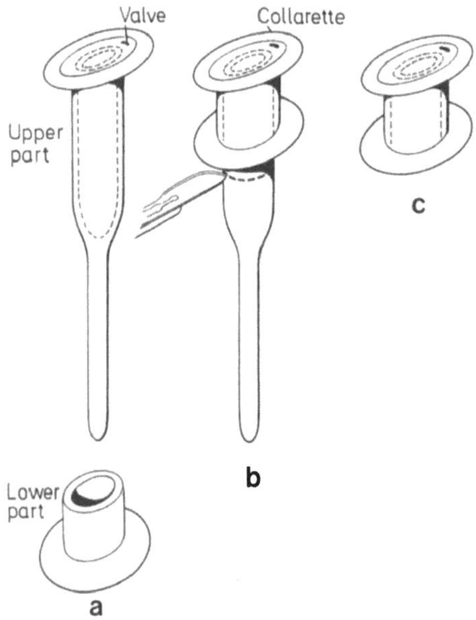

Fig. 1. The prosthesis. The two parts and the aspect of the prosthesis in situ

2. Placement

First of all, we perforate and puncture the tracheo-oesophageal wall with a Reverdin needle. The needle has a strong thread inside which runs as vertically as possible towards the oesophagus. Normally, an endoscopy detects the tip of the needle and the thread just under the shrinking of the Killian mouth. We grasp the thread with forceps and secure it to the thinner end of the higher part of the prosthesis. We drag it through the tracheo-oesophageal wall until it appears on the posterior wall of the tracheostoma. The lower tracheal part is threaded and pushed upwards with the forceps. It is pushed up through the posterior wall of the tracheostoma as high as possible. Afterwards the guide is cut level with the collarette.

3. Results

This experimental study was performed on 36 patients. The voice prostheses are still working today in 19 patients one year later. There was a 51% success rate with the prostheses we had created ourselves. As far as the failures were concerned, 11 patients (i.e., 36%) achieved good oesophageal voice and 5 (i.e., 11%) had no voice at all.

Failure Analysis (16 Cases)

The indications:
1. Neoglottis failure: 12 cases
   3 prosthesis failures due to ejection or incompatibility
2. Shunt failures: 8 cases
   3 prosthesis failures (ejection and extensive granuloma formation).

3. During total laryngectomy: 13 cases
   7 prosthesis failures
   1 patient died in the post-operative period
   3 patients had serious post-operational cicatrization and could not wear the prosthesis
   2 ejections
   1 continuous rotation of the tube with significant aspiration.
4. Placement a long time after laryngectomy
   2 cases of incompatibility (granuloma).

Most of these failures seem to be due to:

1. Incompatibility with the material. Biocompatibility was insufficient and the manufacture imperfect, asperities, valve fixation to a thread which is cut lengthwise.
2. A lack of adaptability between the two pieces of the prosthesis. We think that these problems can be easily avoided.

Phoniatric Results

All of our prosthesis patients are pleased with their voices and do not have deglutition problems. However, they complain about the following:

- Finger occlusion of the tracheostoma during phonation
- Having, in certain cases, to change the prosthesis several times

These complaints make it clear that our prosthesis will have to be improved.

Voice Production

1. Voice Production Waiting Period

Voice production is generally achieved very quickly and ranges from several hours after the first tests to 3–4 days in more difficult cases. The time interval depends on:

a) Learning the reflex motion required to close the tracheostomy or the cannula while not using too much pressure.
b) Sufficient pressure to create an ascending air flow to the posterior wall.

The main reason for voice production failure is the strong pressure created on the tracheostomy or cannula which stops voice production by obstructing the lower tracheal opening of the prostheses. Easy voice production is the right balance between correct finger pressure on the tracheostomy and tracheal air pressure so that the neoglottis (the Killian mouth) can vibrate properly.

2. Intelligibility

Intelligibility is excellent. Articulation is completely retained and does not depend on air refill.

All the phonemas are sonorized. Only one patient complained of not being understood when talking or telephoning.

3. Fluidity, Flow, Modulation

The flow is fluid, i.e., not hacked or stilted. Number counts range from 10–36 but this is not particularly significant because patients count at different speeds. How long patients can pronounce a vowel is more significant. The results vary from 4–20 seconds.

4. Frequency

The frequency of the basic sound varies from person to person. However, it remains constant for any given person even after prosthesis substitute (Fig. 2). This agrees with the fact that sound production is due to mucous vibration of the oesophagus which remains constant in each person. Some sonographs of the vowel "a" show regular impulses with sound patterns which are pleasant to hear. Acoustic analysis indicates that we might be hearing a dysphonic voice (as can occur with a papilloma) and not a prosthetic voice.

Most remarkable of all, our patients can vary their voice frequency so that the majority of them can sing if they want to.

5. Intensity

Our measurements were made by sonometry. The patient was asked to speak normally and then increasingly loudly until he had reached his maximum. Afterwards he had to lower his voice until he had reached the lowest possible level of sonorization. The normal voice intensity produced lay between 70–75 dB for speech and could be easily increased by 10–15 dB. However, it could not be decreased so easily (Fig. 3).

This intensity is sufficient to be heard from one room to another but generally cannot be heard when the patient is in noisy surroundings.

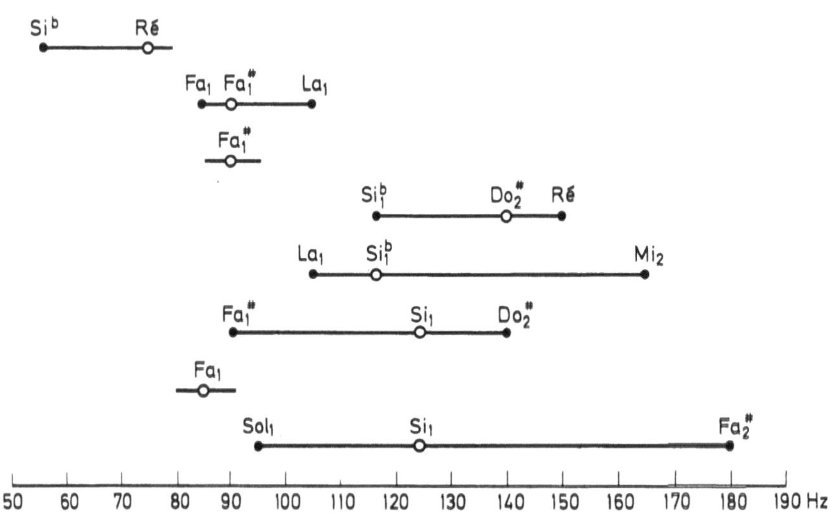

Fig. 2. Study of voice frequencies in our patients

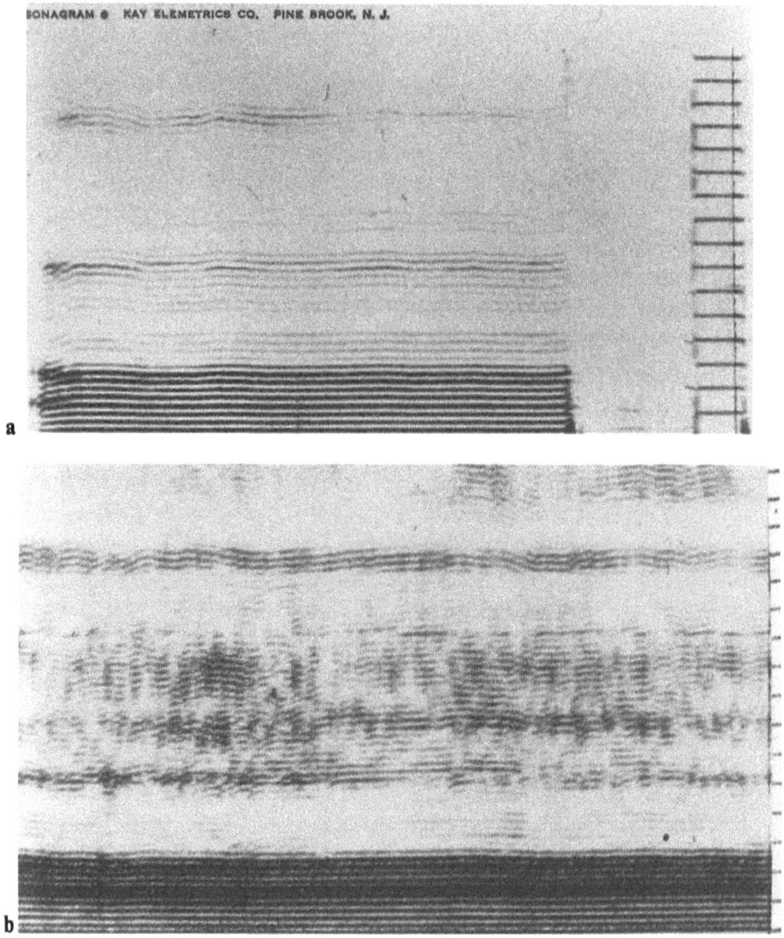

Fig. 3. Sonogramme of a patient with our prosthesis (**b**) compared with a normal one (**a**)

6. Voice Disturbances

Sometimes the tone is "wet" i.e., bubbly because of salivary stasis. This saliva is difficult to swallow because it sticks to the walls and even comes over the sphincter during voice production.

Tracheal Breath Noise

It is sometimes quite difficult to close the tracheostomy and especially the cannula. This resultant noise distresses both the patient and listener for it gives the impression that the patient requires an enormous effort to speak and is straining himself. This is not really the case because his speech is easy under normal circumstances.

Conclusions

Voice production with our prosthesis:
- provides a "human" modulated voice
- retains all intonations
- expresses emotion, affection, cheerfulness, sadness, warmth, coldness. It can also be interrogative or exclamatory etc.
- can start almost immediately
- does not require long and painful training
  This is why it should not be compared with oesophageal speech
- it enables the patient to sing!

The Hypopharyngeal Puncture

H. P. Zenner and I. F. Herrmann[1]

Introduction

By constructing a tracheohypopharyngeal shunt in a patient who has undergone a laryngectomy, intelligible speech can be developed. In order to prevent aspiration, the use of prostheses dates back to the time of the first cancer laryngectomy performed by Billroth in 1873. The device created by Gussenbauer (1874) not only prevented aspiration, but restored the patients voice. 100 years later Mozolewski (this volume, p. 7) developed a miniature valved prosthesis that allowed rapid voice rehabilitation with minimal complications. In 1979 Blom and Singer presented an endoscopic procedure in which a midline tracheoesophageal puncture is performed. They constructed an inexpensive commercially available prosthesis which projects through the upper part of the tracheostoma and is taped to the neck. Furthermore, Herrmann and Kley (1981) as well as Panje (1981) developed silicon valves which could be inserted through the previously formed fistula tract and which are self-contained within the tracheostoma.

Puncture

We have performed an out-patient endoscopic procedure during the last 4 years using a large oesophagoscope. Once the oesophago-hypopharyngeal segment has been reached, the oesophagoscope is rotated so that its mouth is directed towards the dorsal tracheal wall. The point of maximum bulge developing in the tracheostoma indicates the anterior midpoint of the hypopharynx. We designed a puncture needle which is introduced by the surgeon through the posterior tracheal and anterior hypopharyngeal wall along the intended shunt site and into the distal end of the rotated endoscope (Fig. 1a). The puncture site is directed cranially and placed approximately 5 mm from the upper border of the tracheostoma. Subsequently, the puncture needle is removed (Fig. 1b) and replaced by a silicon stent. Figure 1c shows the silicon stent being inserted with an inserter. The stent is retained by an inner retention collar (Fig. 1d). Immediately after puncture, the patient can leave the hospital or office without the stent being visible. The patient is instructed not to remove the silicon stent. Once removed, a stent should be immediately reinserted or the shunt will close within hours.

[1] Universitätsklinik und Poliklinik für Hals-, Nasen- und Ohrenkranke im Kopfklinikum, D-8700 Würzburg.

Speech Restoration Via Voice Prostheses
Edited by I. F. Herrmann

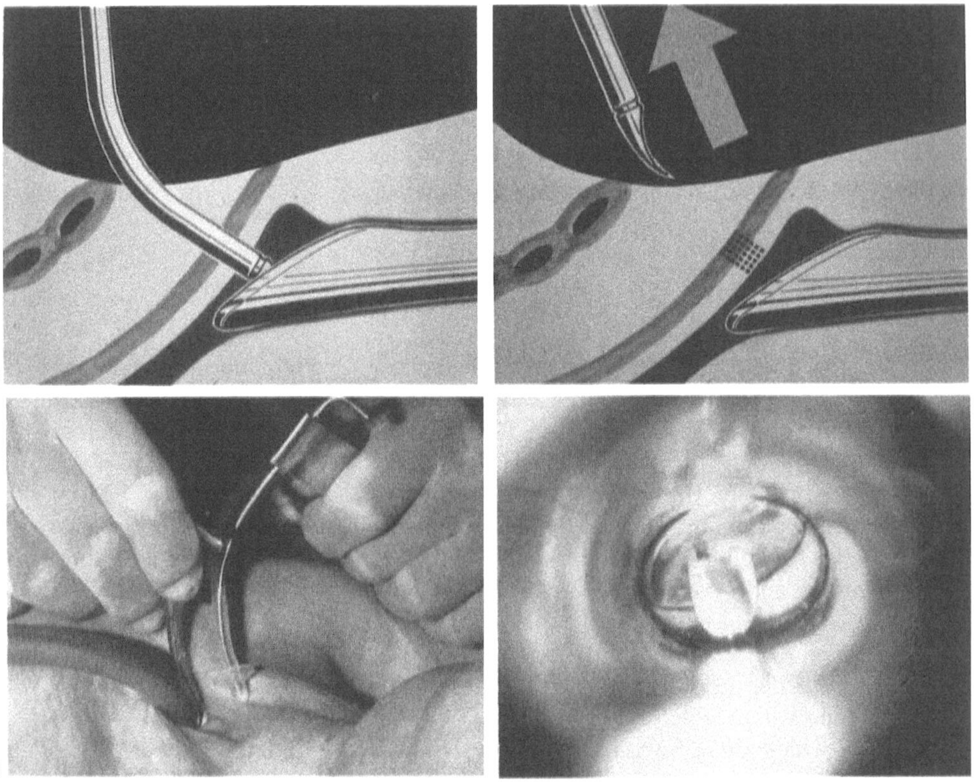

a b c d

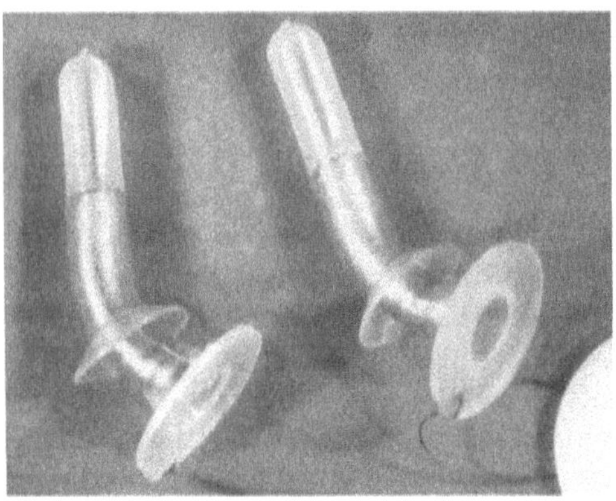

e

Fig. 1. Steps of the secondary tracheopharyngeal (TP) puncture: **a** puncture needle (Koss, Geisenheim, Germany) perforating the posterior tracheal and anterior hypopharyngeal wall thus creating the TP-shunt, **b** removal of puncture needle, **c** insertion of a silicon stent (Koss) into the newly formed shunt, **d** visualization through the rotated oesophagoscope of the inner retention collar of the silicon stent, **e** low pressure valved prostheses (Koss, ESKA-Herrmann type), **f** prosthesis in situ, **g** radiography – prosthesis in situ during "A"-phonation

Voice Prosthesis

2 weeks after puncture, the stent can be removed easily without local anaesthesia and then we insert a low pressure valved prosthesis (ESKA-Herrmann prosthesis, Fa. Koss, Geisenheim, W. Germany) into the newly formed shunt (Fig. 1f). The prosthesis is a convex silicon tube with incorporated inner and outer retention collars (Fig. 1e). Thus, the prosthesis is self-retaining (no cannula required), self-

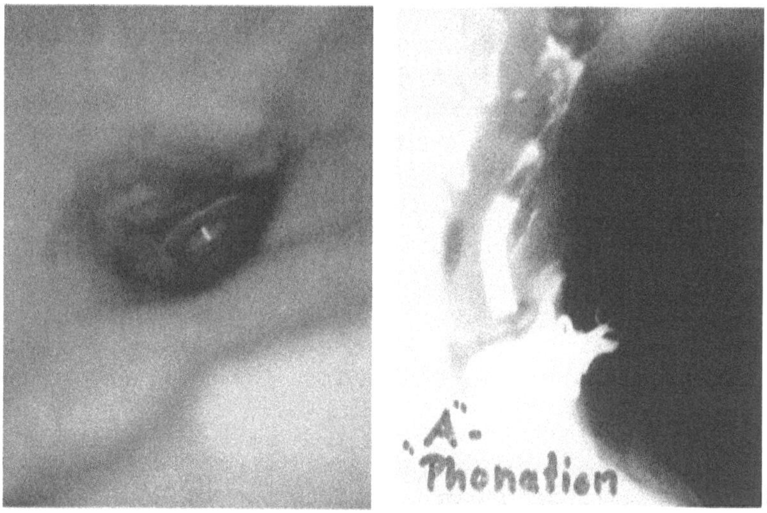

f g

Fig. 1f, g

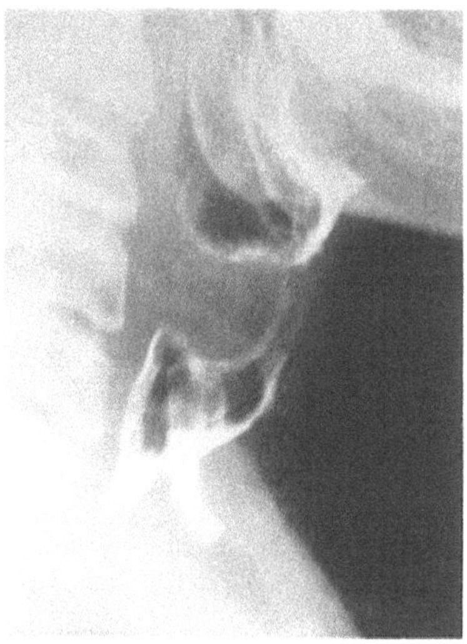

Fig. 2. Contrast radiography of the hypopharynx in a patient without myotomy, dorsal pharyngeal contractile muscle bulk inhibits air flow and diminishes speech production

cleansing (no daily removal required) and situated parallel to the hypopharyngeal mucosa (Fig. 1g).

Results

53 patients have undergone secondary prosthetic voice restoration. Although speech was not perfect it still tended to have the patient's original speech characteristics and dialect patterns. Speech quality was evaluated by the PLT-Test ac-

cording to Zenner (this volume, p. 148) which measures the intelligibility of phonetically balanced monosyllables and sentences. Similar to hearing loss with the speech audiogram, the PLT-test allows to determine the patient's intelligibility loss. The average intelligibility of the linguistic pools on the telephone showed considerable progress compared with oesophageal speech. 60% of the patients with a voice prosthesis developed an intelligibility loss of less than 10%, whereas only 10% of oesophageal speakers belonged to this group. In other words, in contrast to 10% of oesophageal speakers, 60% of the patients with voice prostheses were able to use a telephone.

Failures

However, this figure of 60% still represents a considerable failure of the postlaryngectomy shunt technique. To investigate this question more fully during postoperative visits, intratracheal and intrapharyngeal air pressure, flow and resistance were determined (Herrmann and Kley 1981). Furthermore, pharyngeal mechanics were visualized during speech production by transfistular contrast radiography (Fig. 2). From this it was concluded that voice failures produced severe intrapharyngeal pressure, and reduced mucosal motility created an excessive air flow resistance. Air flow resistance can be decreased by applying lateral and dorsal myotomies during laryngectomy (Hermann and Kley 1981) so that 80% of the laryngectomees demonstrate an intelligibility of less than 10%. 22 patients were punctured following a full course of radiation therapy. Aspiration continued to be a problem in 10 of these cases. The reasons for this were shunt insufficiencies and pharyngeal edemas resulting in leakage. From this experience it is concluded that the secondary shunt technique (in contrast to the primary technique) cannot be recommended for patients who have undergone radiation therapy.

References

Blom ED, Singer MI (1979) Surgical-prosthetic approaches for post-laryngectomy rehabilitation. In: Keith RL, Darley FL (eds) Laryngectomee rehabilitation. College Hill Press, Houston

Gussenbauer C (1874) Über die erste durch Th. Billroth am Menschen ausgeführte Kehlkopf-Exstirpation und die Anwendung eines künstlichen Kehlkopfes. Arch Klin Chir 17:343

Herrmann IF, Kley W (1981) The glottoplasty. Proc XIIth ORL World Congr Budapest

Panje WR (1981) Prosthetic vocal rehabilitation following laryngectomy. Ann Otol Rhinol Laryngol 90:116

Our Experiences with Delayed Primary Voice Rehabilitation

L. P. Löbe [1]

At the ENT clinic of the Martin Luther University in Halle (Saale) about 70 patients with laryngeal cancer are treated annually. Nearly 60% of these required a total laryngectomy. An analysis of the past 10 years proved that 80% of these patients learn to use oesophageal speech and can communicate with other people. Only 22% of these have a good public speaking voice and can use the telephone etc. 20% of them remain "non-speakers".

We have tried to improve the situation by using the vocal fistula of Staffieri. This was not totally successful because of the known problems with aspiration. Since December 1982, we have been using the technique described by Herrmann for our total laryngectomees.

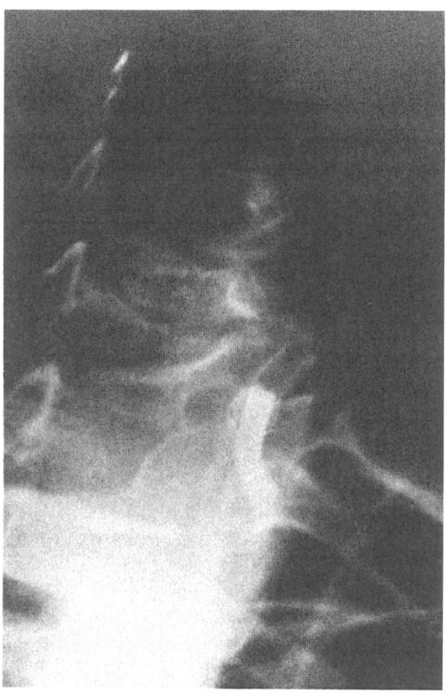

Fig. 1. Correct position of the prosthesis

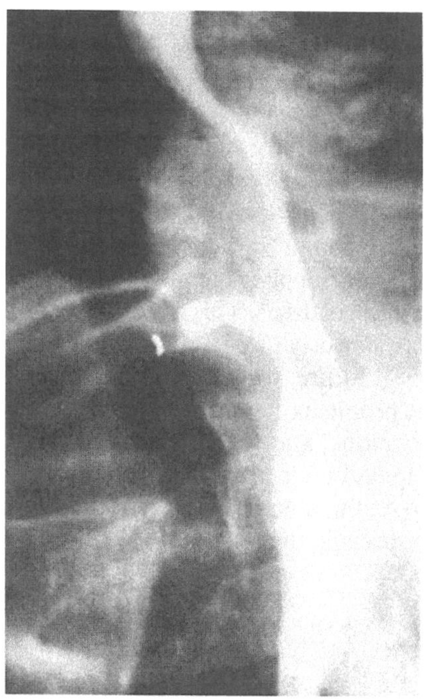

Fig. 2. The prosthesis is turned 180 °

[1] Martin-Luther-Universität, DDR-4020 Halle.

Speech Restoration Via Voice Prostheses
Edited by I. F. Herrmann

We begin with a special skin incision and form a standardized tracheostoma. The posterior wall of the trachea is prepared for tracheo-hypopharyngeal puncture and the myotomy of the muscle constrictor pharyngis is performed. However, the voice prosthesis is not inserted straight away. Instead we wait and see whether the patient is capable of learning traditional oesophageal speech within the next 3–4 months. A tracheo-hypopharyngeal puncture and the insertion of a place retainer follows if oesophageal speech cannot be learned. The Herrmann voice prosthesis is inserted 10 days later.

We have operated 35 patients in this way to date. For 15 of them, it was necessary to perform a tracheo-hypopharyngeal puncture in order to insert the voice prosthesis. We were able to achieve good and quick voice rehabilitation with this procedure in 11 of these 15 patients. This is particularly remarkable as these patients belonged to a negative selection group, i.e., they had only attained rather poor speech performances.

In 4 patients, we had to remove the prostheses after a few weeks or months due to the following problems:

- the patient could not close the tracheostoma with his finger
- too high pressure was needed to take air into the hypopharynx through the prosthesis. This simultaneously resulted in too much side air.
- the prosthesis turned steadily by 180 degrees and caused swallowing difficulties etc. (see Figs. 1, 2)

For the remaining 11 patients, the Herrmann prosthesis was a great success because phonation was immediately possible. There was no need to clean or to change the prosthesis at a later date. Only in 3 cases did we need to renew the button after 2–4 months.

One of our patients has been using the Herrmann prosthesis for 19 months to date.

The steps described above review our current approach. This method represents a compromise between the primary and secondary techniques because primary glottoplasty including myotomy is followed some time later by the insertion of the prosthesis. This is the reason why this procedure is called a delayed primary plastic procedure.

In future, we will continue improving this method and try to solve some of the problems mentioned above. Our work will mainly centre around the operative technique, and the efficiency of the voice button. It will strongly depend on the help and understanding of the speech therapist.

At the moment, we are investigating whether or not this operative technique – especially the myotomy – has any influence on learning traditional oesophageal speech.

Assessment and Management Protocol for Tracheo-Oesophageal "Puncture" Procedures

A. D. CHEESMAN [1], H. HOLDEN [2] and A. PERRY [1]

The early results of tracheo-oesophageal (T-E) puncture at Charing Cross Hospital produced a much lower success rate than reported by the original workers in North America – probably related to the differences in population: e.g., different practices in using radiotherapy; different psycho-social makeup of the patients, etc.

Careful analysis of the problems demonstrated the efficiency of a simple test to detect prosthesis problems. If voice could readily be produced through an open T-E fistula (i.e., *without* prosthesis in situ), and not when the prosthesis is in position, then the prosthesis is at fault. Conversely, if voice is not obtained through the open fistula, the problem generally lies within the functioning of the pharyngo-oesophageal segment.

Considerable development work on the original prostheses has solved many of the early problems: retention; adequate air flow (i.e., low resistance) – reduction of over-fitting and impinging on the posterior oesophageal wall etc. However, comparatively little work has been concentrated on the physiology of alaryngeal speech after T-E "puncture".

Whilst it is fascinating to talk about the different types of voice prostheses now available and the individual aspects of different patients, one question should be asked – viz. "Will the voice prosthesis chosen function in the patient?" It is in order to answer this question that the need for a thorough assessment of each potential should be emphasized. In the Unit at Charing Cross Hospital, a team philosophy prevails. The members of the team consist of the ENT surgeon, radiologist, speech therapist and nursing staff. We believe that, as secondary voice restoration (unlike laryngectomy itself) is not a life-saving procedure, the decision to offer a patient surgical voice restoration should be carefully considered.

The assessments needed obviously have to be adapted to the physical characteristics of the procedure one is choosing and to the characteristics of the prosthesis used. The assessment we use when considering secondary procedures, can be divided into macroscopic and microscopic views. Macroscopic evaluation comes from a detailed case history which the patient is asked to complete, and from a report (where possible) from the referring ENT Surgeon and/or Speech therapist as to the patient's psychological status, e.g., if alcoholism exists. Microscopic

[1] Charing Cross Hospital, Fulham Palace Road, London W6 8RS, Great Britain.
[2] 128 Harley Street, London W1N 1 AH, Great Britain.

Speech Restoration Via Voice Prostheses
Edited by I. F. Herrmann

Table 1. A comparison of phonation techniques

Phonation	Activator	Vibrator	Articulators
Laryngeal	Lungs	Vocal cords	Lips, teeth, tongue etc.
Oesophageal	Oesophagus	P-E segment	As above
T-E "puncture"	Lungs	P-E segment	As above

evaluation focusses externally on anatomical and physiological considerations. The site of stoma/trachea; sensitivity of stoma/tracheal area and internally – the viability of the P-E segment.

If one compares laryngeal, oesophageal and tracheo-oesophageal (T-E) (Table 1) voice it can be seen that the vibratory site for both oesophageal and T-E voice is the same; viz: the P-E segment. It is for this reason that one needs to ascertain that the reason for non-attainment of oesophageal voice is not a failure in the activity of the P-E segment. If so, this may also impede the success of T-E voice unless the problem is first attended to.

At Charing Cross Hospital, we use mainly the Blom-Singer and Panje procedures, so our assessments include examination of the activity of the P-E segment. If we were using, for example, an external Reed fistula, e.g., Shedd's Reed fistula prosthesis – we would not need to be so concerned with the status of the P-E segment as it would not be a source of vibration (Shedd and Bakamjian 1972).

The Charing Cross Hospital evaluation of patients' voicing mechanism relies predominantly on videofluroscopy. A team including ENT Surgeon, radiologist, speech pathologist and video technician meets once a month and assesses 6–8 new

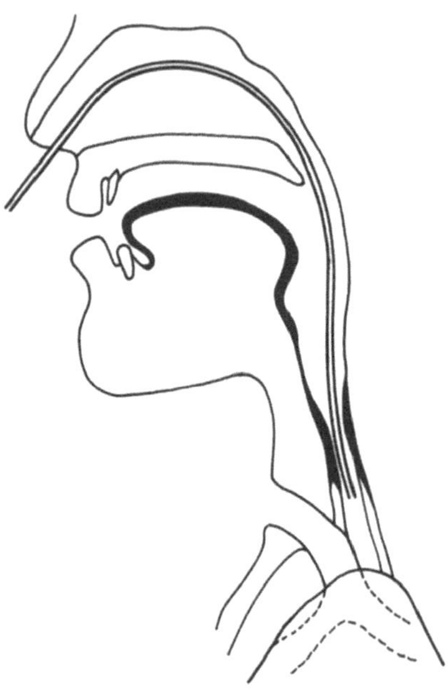

Fig. 1. Taub airblowing test to show position of catheter

Table 2

		Hypertonicity		
		/	\	
Hypotonic	Good oesophageal speakers	Hypertonic	Spasm	Stricture
→	→	→	→	

Table 3. Hypotonic patients

Barium swallow	Phonation	Air insufflation
Fast motility Pharynx – oesophagus opens	No P-E segment visible	Whispery/no phonation. Better with digital pressure i.e. *sl. positive*

patients per clinic. The 3 parts of the videofluroscopy are: A Barium swallow, attempted phonation, and an air insufflation test.

The Barium swallow will often detect physical problems which may have affected the patient's ability to acquire oesophageal voice, e.g., hiatus hernia, and/or high or low mucosal pouches. These factors may account for failed oesophageal speech but will be irrelevant to T-E success. During the swallow, we note motility time and the outline of the oral cavity, pharynx, and oesophagus during deglutition.

"Phonation" consists of asking the patient to attempt to count from 1 to 10 and noting any oesophageal/pharyngeal movements as well as any air mobility within the oesophagus and/or pharynx. We also note the quality/type of voice achieved (if any).

Air insufflation, as described by other speakers, consists of a transnasal 14 FG catheter being inserted into the top of the oesophagus through the P-E segment and externally blowing air passively into the oesophagus (Fig. 1).

The type and quality of phonation achieved during this act is noted. The 50 patients we have looked at during the first 9 months of this project seem to fall into 4 categories along a spectrum: (1) hypotonic, (2) good oesophageal speakers, (3) overall hypertonicity subdivided into hypertonic, and (4) "spasm". A 5th category of stricture patients also existed (Table 2).

The hypotonic patient reacts as follows under videofluroscopy (Table 3): On swallowing, the motility time is fast and the whole of the pharynx to oesophagus clearly opens. During phonation, no P-E segment is visible. On air insufflation, whispery or non-phonation results unless digital pressure is applied – when the voice becomes much louder/clearer.

Good oesophageal speakers react as follows (Table 4): On swallowing, fast motility time is seen. On phonation, a good oesophageal air reservoir and a clear P-E segment are visible. On air insufflation testing, good voicing is achieved.

The "stricture" patients have quite different results (Table 5): On swallowing, a clear hold up to Barium is seen – there is little or no dilation of the pharynx and oesophagus and slow motility time results. They usually report swallowing problems (dysphagia). On phonation, little or no air enters the oesophagus and no

Table 4. Good oesophageal speakers

Barium swallow	Phonation	Air Insufflation
Fast motility Pharynx – oesophagus opens	One P-E segment Good oesophageal air reservoir	Good voice – as own, i.e. *positive*

Table 5. "Stricture" patients

Barium swallow	Phonation	Air insufflation
Slow motility Hold up to Ba. little/no dilation Reports dysphagia	Little/no air in oesophagus	No voice achieved Oesophagus inflates but no P-E opening visible, i.e. *negative*

Table 6. Hypertonic patients

Barium swallow	Phonation	Air insufflation
Sl. narrowing often visible in pharynx but this *dilates*	One tight *or* two P-E segments visible. Good oesophageal air reservoir. Poor voice	Better voice on *gentle* airblowing, i.e. *positive*

Table 7. Spasm

Barium swallow	Phonation	Air insufflation
Slight narrowing in pharyngooesophageal area. Often visible, *but dilates*	Very tight P-E segment. Oesophageal air reservoir poor. Very poor/no voice often pharyngeal	No voice achieved. Oesophagus fills; P-E segment very tight and then explosively releases i.e. *negative*

Table 8. To achieve successful voicing

Hypertonicity			
Hypotonic	Hypertonic	Spasm	Stricture
Needs digital pressure	Myotomy? *or* low pressure valve	Myotomy	Surgery to relieve stricture or Bouginage

voicing is heard. On air insufflation, no voice is heard. The oesophagus may or may not inflate, but there appears to be no P-E segment opening/vibrating.

We have now sub-divided the overall "hypertonicity" group into two – those who are "hypertonic" and those who show total "spasm", as described by Singer and Blom (1983). This is a group which presents problems on air insufflation testing and where we feel videofluroscopy is invaluable in assessment. They react as

Table 9. Failed oesophageal speakers

	Hypotonic	Good oesophageal voice	Hypertonicity		Stricture
			Hypertonic	Spasm	
Barium swallow	Oesophagus – pharynx dilates. Fast motility	Pharynx – oesophagus opens. Fast motility	Slight narrowing in tract visible but dilates	Slight narrowing in tract. Dilates	Hold up to Barium. Little/no dilation. Reports dysphagia. Slow motility
Phonation	No P-E segment visible	One P-E segment visible. Good oesophageal air reservoir	One tight or 2 P-E segments visible. Poor voice.	Very tight P-E segment. Oesophageal air is good. Very poor/ no voice	Little/no air penetrates oesophagus
Air insufflation test	Whispery/no phonation	Good voice – as own	Better voice on *gentle* airblowing	No voice achieved. Very tight P-E segments. Explosively releases	No voice – oesophagus inflates but no P-E opening
	Slight positive	*Positive*	*Positive*	*Negative*	*Negative*

follows (Table 6): The hypertonic patient shows dilation of the pharynx and oesophagus on swallowing, despite the presence of a slight narrowing being often visible at the pharyngo-oesophageal juncture.

On attempted phonation, these patients often show *two* clear segments vibrating *or* they may show one tight (vibrating) P-E segment with a good oesophageal reservoir underneath. Poor voice is heard. On air insufflation, they may achieve good voice (i.e., a positive result) on *gentle* air blowing but when the air is blown too forcefully, they may resist phonation and go into "spasm".

The group we call "true" spasm reacts as follows (Table 7): On Barium swallowing, there may be a narrow area in the pharynx, which dilates well. On attempted phonation, these patients show a very tight P-E segment with a variable amount of air in the oesophagus. No voice is produced. On air insufflation testing, there is either no voice at all, or a sudden explosive sound as the P-E segment releases explosively, i.e., this is a negative air insufflation test result.

How then does the management of the patients vary, according to the results achieved?

The "Bottom Line" is as follows (Table 8): We feel that each patient will fall into one of these groups within a spectrum. For positive results on T-E procedures, the following are necessary:

- The hypotonic patient will need digital pressure to achieve good voicing results.
- The stricture patients will need surgery to remove the constriction.
- The overall "hypertonicity" group will vary according to the amount of tone present:

Table 10. Breakdown of patients within each group: $N=50$

Good oesophageal speakers	8
Hypotonic	9
Hypertonic	17
Spasm	15
Stricture	1

The "spasm" group will certainly need a pharyngo-oesophageal myotomy to relieve the muscular spasm prior to T-E puncture being undertaken.

But the "hypertonic" group may be managed either by a pre-puncture myotomy or by selecting a low resistance voice prosthesis to enable the flow of air to be smooth and continuous without a sudden "burst" of air being emitted into the oesophagus, as happens with the higher pressure prostheses. This process improves with learning therapy.

This has been an effective choise for a number of our patients within this "hypertonic" group who have refused to have a myotomy but who have wanted a T-E procedure. The summarized assessments are shown in Table 9.

The number of patients who have fallen into each category, from a total of 50, is shown in Table 10.

We feel it is important that accurate assessment of the patients and allocation into these groups is made, in order to delineate the two groups within the overall "hypertonicity" category. It may be that myotomy is not always necessary in these patients, if the hypertonicity is below a certain level. Currently, we are undertaking objective measurements of air pressure and flow within this group of patient. This will hopefully give us clear "cut off" points within the two groups and enable the decision for myotomy surgery to be taken more scientifically.

Surgical Aspects of Tracheo-Oesophageal Puncture

Puncture Technique

The actual puncture technique has been simplified by the use of a flexible 14 F.G. trocar. The trocar has been constructed from a 14 F.G. diameter teflon rod with a sharpened metal point at one end, and a threaded insert at the other end to which is attached a 14 F.G. plastic catheter. The puncture site in the tracheo-oesophageal wall is clearly demonstrated by transillumination from an unmodified distally-lit bronchoscope passed down the pharynx. The trocar is easily passed through the party-wall into the lumen of the bronchoscope which is then withdrawn with the trocar within its lumen, drawing the catheter through the fistula. The catheter is then transferred to the nasal cavity, and left in place for 48 hours.

Originally, great care was taken to distinguish between the Blom-Singer and Panje puncture sites. However, we now realize that since we have used one-strap Blom-Singer prostheses this is not too important. The actual site of puncture is now determined by the anatomy of the stoma and planned to allow ease of insertion of the prostheses by the patient. Prosthetic insertion is generally performed after 48 hours when the fistula tract has stabilised.

Surgical Problems/Considerations

1. Stoma

Ideally, the stoma needs to be about 1.5 cm in diameter. This allows easy manipulation of the prosthesis but the stoma should not be so big as to prevent finger occlusion. Many of our patients had small stomas on presentation which needed surgical correction. Several patients also developed stenosis following "puncture", presumably the result of scarring in irradiated tissue. After trying many different ways of enlarging the stoma, we found the most effective was a Y-V advancement of skin into the inferior lip of the stoma. This left the posterior puncture site untouched by stoma revision surgery.

2. Pharyngeal Strictures

The presence of strictures at the site of pharyngeal repair is not uncommon and generally interferes with surgical speech rehabilitation. Such strictures must be corrected surgically either by resection and resuture or by the transposition of skin into the pharynx. Both methods produce good voice with subsequent tracheo-oesophageal puncture.

3. Crico-Pharyngeal Spasm

Pharyngeal spasm, as indicated previously, must be corrected by crico-pharyngeal myotomy, and we would agree with Singer and Blom that a long myotomy is necessary. It is our practice to suture the divided muscle layer away from the line of incision to prevent reformation of the muscle layer by scar tissue.

4. Infection

Two patients developed a localized infection of the party-wall following puncture. Removal of the catheter and systemic antibiotics rapidly resolved the infection and subsequent re-puncture was uneventful.

5. Sterno-Mastoid Tenotomy

Division of the tendons of the sternomastoid muscles results in a flatter contour to the peri-stomal area and allows better adhesion of the tracheostoma valve housing in many patients.

Surgical Reconstruction of the Pharynx

Careful analysis, comparing the method of surgical repair of the pharynx at laryngectomy with subsequent voice production using videofluroscopy, has provided very useful information. This information establishes the indications for an ideal pharyngeal repair at laryngectomy to produce the best possible environment for voice production – whether this is using oesophageal or tracheo-oesophageal "puncture" voice. The most obvious lesson we have learned from our videofluroscopy studies is that a multi-layer muscular closure, as traditionally practised to prevent pharyngeal fistula formation, is most inappropriate for subsequent voice rehabilitation either by oesophageal or fistula speech. This finding is the complete opposite of the classic study by Simpson et al. 1972, and we think that our results may have been influenced by the use of pre-operative radiotherapy in all our cases. Most cases with this type of pharyngeal repair have required pharyngeal myotomy before acquiring both good oesophageal and fistula speech.

We are now using videofluroscopy to study various different modifications of pharyngeal repair. Although the work is still in its early stages, it is already apparent that the following techniques produce beneficial results:

a) Pharyngeal myotomy at the time of laryngectomy is of prime importance.
b) Another satisfactory variation is to suture the inferior constrictor fibres to the supra-hyoid muscles, above and not across the pharyngeal closure.

This provides good pharyngeal tone but does not constrict the pharyngeal lumen. The technique of merely closing the pharyngeal mucosa without any muscle suture results in a hypotonic pharynx. Digital pressure is then necessary for adequate vocalisation. The use of transposed skin or abdominal viscera generally results in a satisfactors pharynx for the generation of fistula speech. However, videofluroscopy studies show a generally hypotonic pharynx in such cases. It is our hope to be able to advise on an appropriate technique for pharyngeal repair within the near future, which will result in an active pharyngo-oesophageal segment without excessive spasm.

Acknowledgements. To Mrs. Rhona Ward for her excellent typing skills and to the Department of Medical Illustration at Charing Cross Hospital for their assistance in preparation of this manuscript and in the provision of illustrations.

References

Perry A et al. (1982) A modification of the Blom-Singer-valve for restoration of voice after laryngectomy. J.L.O. Vol. XCVI, No. 11

Shedd Dp, Bakamjian V (1972) Am J Surg 124:510

Chapter 2 Experimental Research Regarding the Function and Handling of Voice Prostheses

Physical Aspects of Tracheo-Oesophageal Shunt Prostheses (Pressure – Flow Measurements of a Model Prosthesis)

F. Schön [1]

Prostheses for speech restoration are part of a very complex physiological system. One component of this system, the prosthesis itself and its interaction with the trachea, can be studied in vitro. Moreover, its behavior can be understood on the basis of aerodynamics. A mathematical model of this system is not only extremely helpful in the area of prosthesis design, but also improves our understanding of the more important interactions with the oesophageal system.

1. Experimental Design

Because the soft lips of the silicon ESKA-Herrmann prostheses cannot be fixed in a definite way, model prostheses were made: Stiff brass lips (15 mm long) were connected to a brass tube (3 mm inner diameter; 30 mm long) via a short elastic tube. Different prosthesis materials can be simulated easily by varying the length of the elastic tube. The model prostheses are inserted into a wider tube (19 mm diameter) which serves as a substitute for the trachea. The pressure in this wider tube is monitored by a pressure transducer. Thus the pressure measured is directly related to the pressure needed by a patient to overcome the opposition of the prosthesis in situ. Air flow was measured in front of the wider tube with a highly sensitive differential pressure transducer via a flow element. The transducer signals are fed to a Commodore personal computer, displayed on the CRT, and stored on a floppy disk.

2. Modelling of Characteristics

For the air flow from the trachea through the prosthesis one can distinguish three regions: There is an entrance region of the air to the prosthesis, followed by a tubular section of the prosthesis, and finally a valve part. The pressure loss in the tubular part of the prosthesis is caused by friction, whereas the pressure drop caused by the other two parts mainly reflects the increase in dynamic pressure due to the narrowing of the cross-section.

[1] Universitätsklinik und Poliklinik für Hals-, Nasen- und Ohrenkranke im Kopfklinikum, D-8700 Würzburg.

Speech Restoration Via Voice Prostheses
Edited by I. F. Herrmann

a) Resistance of the Tubular Section

The tubular part of the prosthesis can be treated as a smooth pipe of length l and diameter d. Using the resistance formula of Darcy Weiskopf, we have:

$p_1 - p_2 = f\,(l/d) * \varrho v^2/2.$

The friction factor f for turbulent flow in a smooth pipe is given by the Blasius formula: $\log(f) = -0.25 \log(Re) - 0.5$. Re stands for the Reynolds number, p for pressure, v for velocity and ϱ for density. The flow is turbulent for Reynolds numbers > 2320, corresponding to a flow of 82 ml/s for the pipe in question. As this pressure drop never contributes to more than about 20% of the total pressure drop, we also used this formula to correct frictional pressure loss in the laminar region.

b) Air Entrance Effects

The Bernoulli equation describes the dynamic pressure increase caused by the narrowing at the prosthesis inlet. However, as the air stream contracts to a smaller diameter than that of the prosthesis lumen, eddies are produced. These eddies dissipate mechanical energy, so a loss term has to be taken into account:

$p_1 + \varrho v_1^2/2 = p_2 + \varrho v_2^2/2 + p_{loss}.$

We found $p_{loss} = 0.45\,\varrho v_2^2/2$ for our sharply cut tube, which agrees well with the resistance coefficients given in the literature. The characteristics of the tube, including air entrance effects and frictional losses, are shown in Fig. 1.

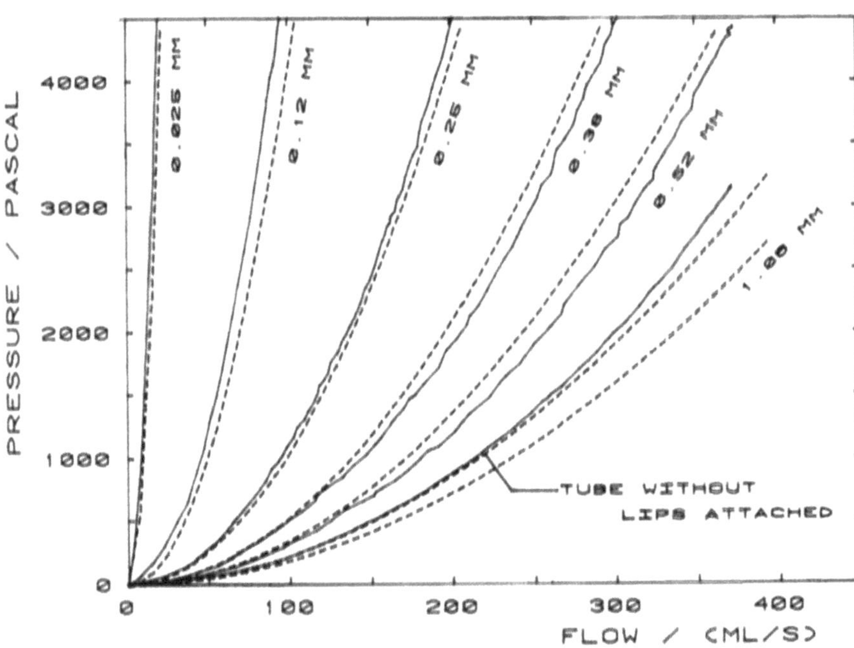

Fig. 1. Pressure – flow characteristics of a model prosthesis for various set lip opening widths. The width of the cleft is measured in the middle of the outlet. Experimental (—), theoretical (---) results

c) Valve Resistance

Even if the valve lips are only opened slightly, the air is subjected to another sudden narrowing. In this case the Bernoulli equation has to be modified again. This is not only to compensate for pressure loss but also for the smaller efflux due to stream contraction. 3, 4 and 5 mm diameter model prostheses were investigated. When the lips are almost completely closed, the effective area is decreased to 63% of the geometrical slit area between the lips, whereas the pressure is increased by a factor of 2.5. The loss term, $p_{loss} = 0.3\ \varrho v_1^2/2$, becomes important for moderately opened lips. The air stream does not expand into the cross-section of the lips but builds up into a jet. Thus, dynamic energy of the stream is wasted outside of the valve and cannot be won back to compensate the transdevice pressure drop. Finally, the influence of widely-opened lips becomes negligible and the characteristics are approximately equal to that of a tube without lips.

A transition region exists where the transdevice pressure is slightly lower in a prosthesis than in a tube. In this region, there is not too good an approximation. However, we obtained reasonable results by substituting the pressure drop of the prosthesis with that of a tube, if the pressure declined more than the tube. Figure 1 shows the total pressure drop as measured and computed for set lip opening widths.

d) Pressure – Flow Characteristics

In order to compute the pressure – flow characteristics of a prosthesis, a relationship between the outlet width and the transdevice flow rate needs to be derived.

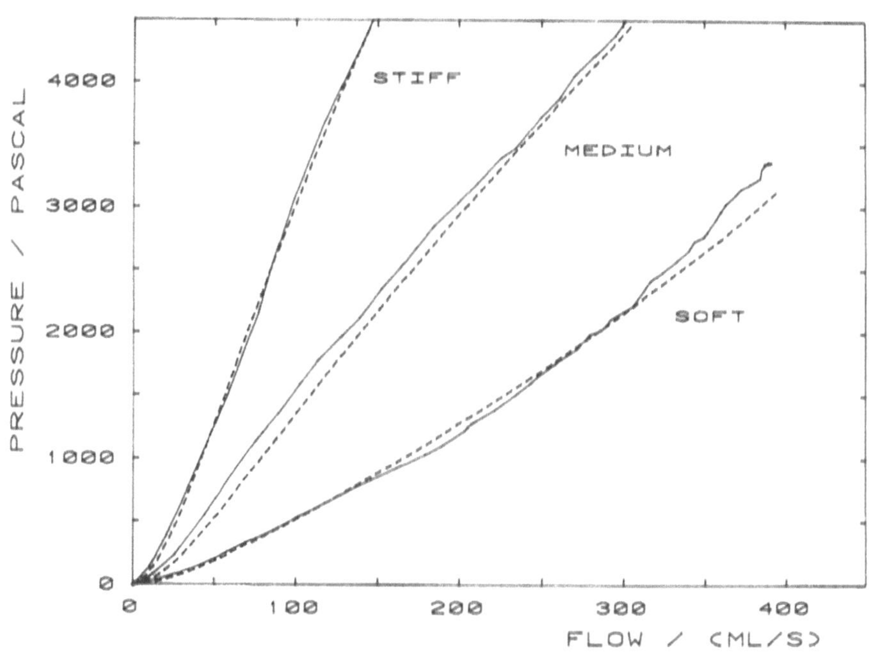

Fig. 2. Pressure – flow characteristics of a model prosthesis. Three different materials, soft, medium, and stiff, are simulated. Experimental (—), theoretical (---) results

We measured the width of the lip opening with increasing flow using the linear approximations below for further computations. Three different prosthesis materials were simulated:

cleft width/mm = 0.0016 *flow/(ml/s) + 0.225 ("soft lips")
cleft width/mm = 0.0009 *flow/(ml/s) + 0.125 ("medium stiff lips")
cleft width/mm = 0.00065*flow/(ml/s) + 0.075 ("stiff lips").

The results are shown in Fig. 2. The "soft lips" results closely resemble the characteristics of a tube. They form a concave curve reflecting an increasing pressure proportional to the square of the flow caused by the dynamic pressure term in the Bernoulli equation. The "stiff lips" produce another set of characteristics and a convex curve is found. In this case, the valve part of the prosthesis is the dominant characteristic. According to the Bernoulli equation, the pressure will still increase with the square of the flow. However, it also decreases with the square of the width of the lip opening. If one assumes that the opening of the prosthesis lip can be described by a torsional spring constant as with Moon et al. (1983), the width increases proportionally to inner prostheses pressure. These combined relations show pressure $\propto$ flow $^{2/3}$ as given by Moon et al. (1983). The graph of this equation is convex and resembles that obtained with the "stiff lips" model. By chance, the prostheses of Blom and Singer and some of the ESKA-Herrmann prostheses show linear flow – pressure characteristics which are almost similar to the "medium" model.

Reference

Moon JB et al. (1983) Evaluation of Blom-Singer tracheoesophageal puncture prostheses performance. J Speech Hearing Research 26:459–464

In Vitro Experiments Using Valve Prostheses

P. KARSCHAY [1]

The prerequisite for effortless tracheo-pharyngeal speech is low flow resistance.

First, we tested the various qualities of a conventional voice prosthesis (Singer and Blom 1980) which influence flow resistance.

Figure 1 shows the variable prosthesis parameters:

- the inside diameter
- the length of the slit
- the length of the prosthesis
- the position of the slit
- the prosthesis material
- lateral or coaxial insufflation of an old Blom-Singer prosthesis.

Our experiments show that flow resistance primarily depends on the slit length and diameter of the prosthesis. Figure 1 summarizes the results: a mere 1 mm reduction of the internal prosthesis diameter more than doubles the pressure under constant flow. A 2 mm decrease in slit length, i.e., from 8 mm to 6 mm doubles the flow resistance. There is, however, only a 10% change in flow resistance:

- when the length of the prosthesis is reduced by 5 mm
- when the valve lip is displaced laterally from the median plane

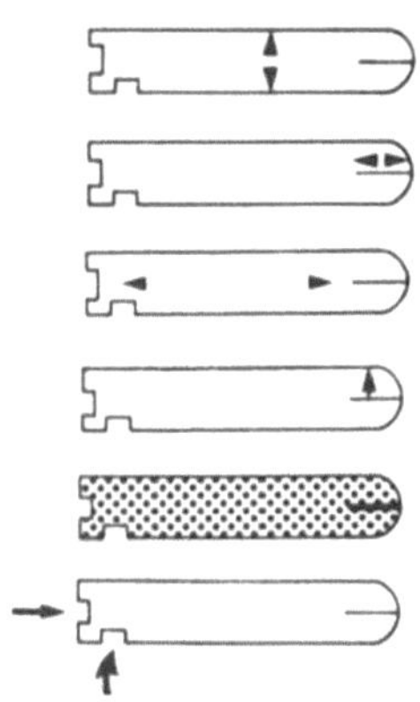

scheme	explanation	change of resistance
	inner diameter by 1 mm	more than 100 p.c.
	slit length by 2 mm	100 p.c.
	length of prosthesis reduced by 5 mm	10 p.c.
	lateral slitted prosthesis	10 p.c.
	silicon / metal tube	10 p.c.
	change of the direction of insufflation	10 p.c.

Fig. 1. The conventional Blom-Singer voice prosthesis and flow resistance

[1] Universitätsklinik und Poliklinik für Hals-, Nasen- und Ohrenkranke im Kopfklinikum, D-8700 Würzburg.

Speech Restoration Via Voice Prostheses
Edited by I. F. Herrmann

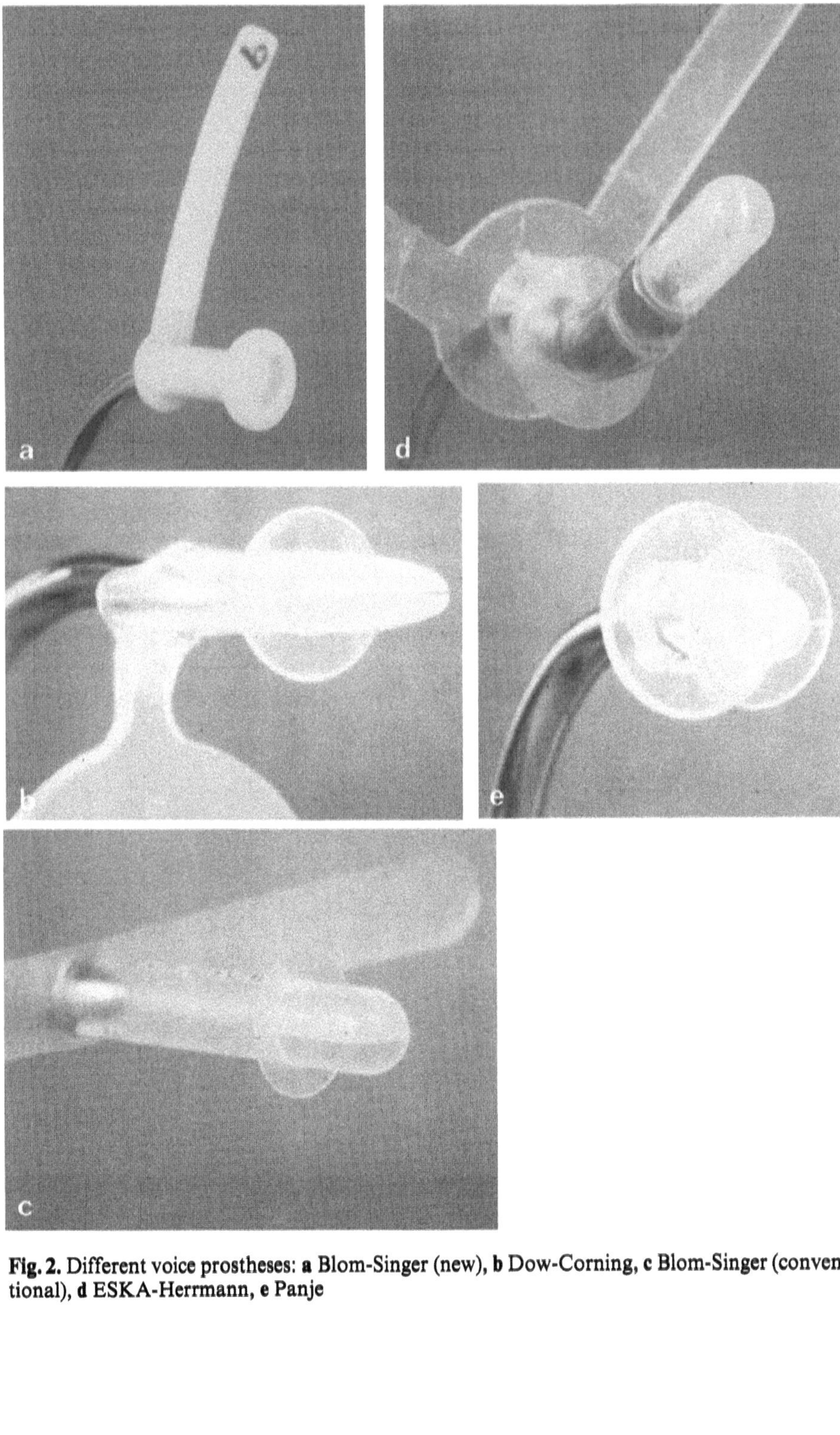

Fig. 2. Different voice prostheses: **a** Blom-Singer (new), **b** Dow-Corning, **c** Blom-Singer (conventional), **d** ESKA-Herrmann, **e** Panje

- when a metal tube is used instead of coarse-grained silicon
- when insufflation is modified.

Not very many prostheses used to be produced with a larger internal diameter. This is because food passing throught the pharynx used to be an impediment. The prosthesis slit can only be enlarged, if valve function is not impaired. Since 1980, various different types of voice prostheses have been developed. They differ from each other both in some of the above parameters and in the way the valve is used:

- Fig. 2a: the new Blom-Singer prosthesis with a little silicon plate for a valve (inventor's own data).
- Fig. 2b: the Dow-Corning prosthesis (Henley-Cohn 1981) with an oval lumen when seen in cross-section. The pharyngeal end has a horizontal slit for a valve and is conic.
- Fig. 2c: the old Singer-Blom voice prosthesis (1980) which also has a horizontal valve slit.
- Fig. 2d: a valve prosthesis developed in Würzburg (Herrmann 1983). A metal tube serves as a directional stabilizer in the hypopharynx. Two silicon discs keep the prosthesis in the shunt. The valve consists of a vertical slit.
- Fig. 2e: the voice button (Panje 1981) with a radial slit.

All five of these prostheses have different flow-pressure curves (Fig. 3). The ordinate shows the flow in ml/s and the abscissa the pressure in Pascals. The loop-like shape of the curves is due to the elastic after-effect i.e., the so-called hysteresis of the prosthesis material: A constant flow increase raises pressure more than a constant decrease.

The resistance figures for the individual prostheses, which are obtained by dividing pressure by flow, show the way air passes through the prosthesis (Table 1).

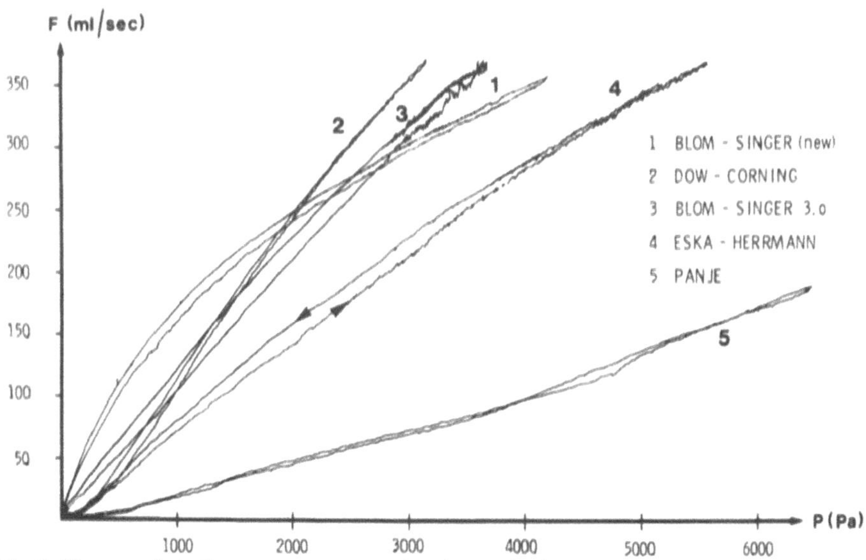

Fig. 3. Characteristic flow-pressure curve of each prosthesis

Table 1. Resistance figures for each prosthesis

Model of prosthesis	Resistance Pa/(ml/s) (for F = 100 ml/s)
Blom-Singer (new)	4
Dow-Corning	9.5
Blom-Singer 3.0	10
ESKA-Herrmann	13.5
Panje	40.5

When insufflating a Panje prosthesis at 100 ml per second, for example, the resistance is approximately 4 times higher than that in a Dow-Corning prosthesis.

Finger pressure on the tracheostoma during phonation can move the voice prosthesis closer to the spine. In radiological experiments, we insufflated barium sulphate dust into the pharynx via an old Blom-Singer prosthesis. We found that the prosthesis can be displaced cranially or caudally by the above-mentioned contact with surrounding tissue. Mechanical pressure upon the slit impedes the exhalation of air in each case.

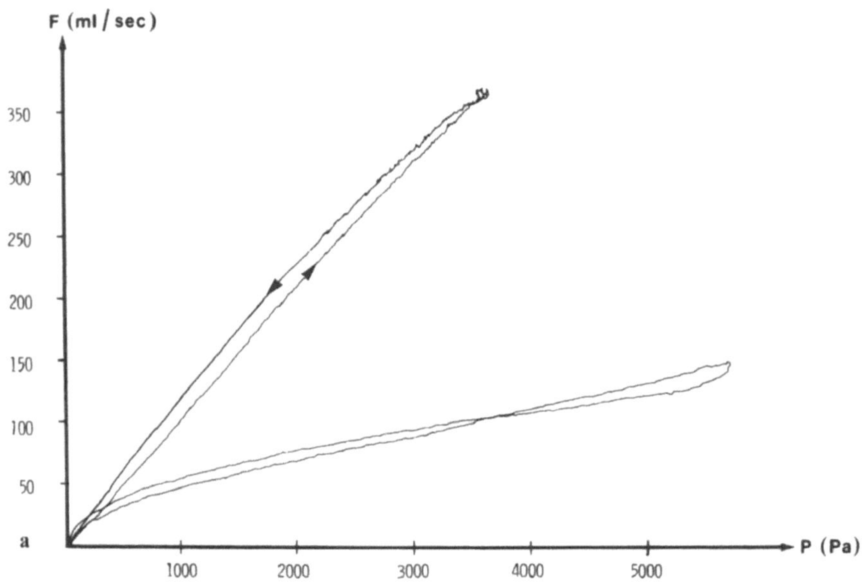

a

	resistance Pa / ml/sec (for F = loo ml/sec.)	
	no contact	contact
BLOM - SINGER 3.o	lo	34

b

Fig. 4. a Characteristic flow-pressure curve of a Blom-Singer prosthesis with (*lower loop*) and without (*upper loop*) membrane contact. **b** The resultant resistances

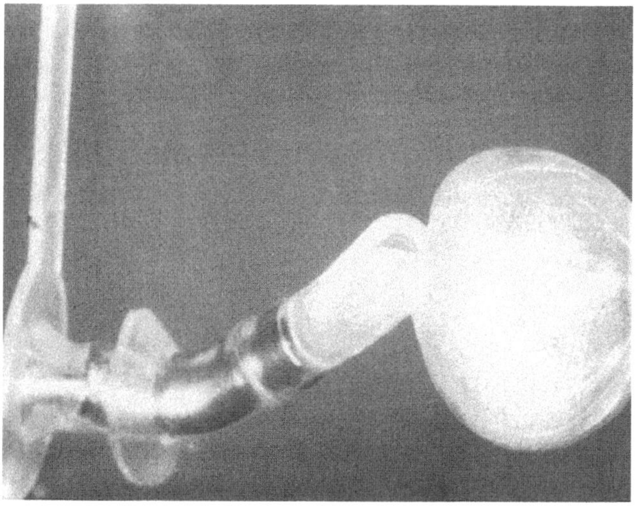

a

	resistance Pa/ml/sec. (for F = 100 ml/sec.)	
	no contact	contact
ESKA - HERRMANN	13.5	5

b

Fig. 5. a The vertical slit of an Eska-Herrmann prosthesis opens on contact. **b** The resultant resistance figures with and without contact

On the basis of these observations, we drew the characteristic flow-pressure curve of different prosthesis types in vitro with and without simulated tissue contact: Figure 4 a shows the characteristic flow-pressure curve of the old Blom-Singer voice prosthesis with (upper loop) and without (lower loop) contact. In this case, flow resistance roughly tripled (Fig. 5 b). A decrease in flow resistance due to contact with surrounding tissue might also be possible. The model in Fig. 5 a shows how a vertical slit opens on contact. We found that the resistance decreases to just above half its original level (Fig. 5 b).

All these experiments were repeated using simulated human mucosal contact. Corresponding results were duly found. The short pharyngeal end of the new Blom-Singer voice prosthesis is unlikely to produce greater air flow resistance with wall contact. Low resistance voice prostheses are only partly responsible for easy phonation. Perhaps contact between the pharyngeal end of the prosthesis and the surrounding tissue considerably influences flow resistance. Furthermore, a valve prosthesis patient has to overcome total resistance which, among other things, includes the resistance of the pharyngeal constrictor muscles. Apart from trying to design low resistance voice prostheses, we must try to find surgical ways of creating low resistance and a vibratile upper digestive tract.

References

Henley-Cohn J (1981) „How I do it" – Head and neck: a targeted problem and its solution. New technique for insertion of laryngeal prosthesis. Laryngoscope 91:1957–1959

Herrmann IF (1983) Surgical speech restoration using a voice prosthesis. Arch Otorhinolaryng

Panje WR (1981) Prosthetic voice rehabilitation following laryngectomy. The voice button. Ann Otol Rhinol Laryngol 90:116–20

Singer MI, Blom ED (1980) An endoscopic technique for restoration of voice after laryngectomy. Ann Otol Rhinol Laryngol 89:529–533

Wear and Tear on the Silicon of Valve Prostheses in the Upper Digestive Tract – A Study Using Electron Microscope Scanning

I. F. Herrmann [1], G. Poschet [2] and J. Zöhren [2]

Valve prostheses in the digestive tract are subject to the effects of food, drink, and saliva. Moreover, they are under permanent mechanical stress caused by the distension and contraction of the surrounding muscles. In other words, they are under mechanical, chemical, and bacteriological attack. Extended observation indicates that deposits collect on the silicon surface which affect the elasticity of the plastic. Our studies are researching these changes in the plastic. Their aim is to develop a more resistant plastic which remains compatible with the digestive tract.

Electronic Microscope Scanning (EMS)

EMS investigations of valve prosthesis surfaces analyse the deposits and their effects on the material. First, the surfaces are sputtered with a sputter coater and observed as well as photographed at various magnifications. The μ marker (white strip + number) shows the magnitude on the bottom right hand edge of the photographs printed below.

Newly-manufactured prostheses have a smooth surface (Fig. 1). However, a film can be seen on the prosthesis surface only an hour after insertion in the patient (Fig. 2). Fungus colonization begins after a day and spreads in reticular fashion. One week later, bacteria can be detected in the network of the fungi culture (Fig. 3). The deposition of amorphous food particles then follows. After two to three weeks, the film on the silicon cannot be detached. Using silicon sections of the valve prostheses, it was possible to prove that hyphae penetrate the silicon and thus make a firm anchorage possible. Fungus colonization can be detected on the outside of the valve lips and somewhat later on their inside. Thus the deposits advance slowly from the outside to the rims of the valve and can finally lead to valve insufficiency. As the coating is kept soft in the moist region of the digestive tract, it hardly impairs vocal fold function. The coatings seen after months or years of wear vary to a remarkable extent when viewed under the scanning electron microscope.

The deposits proved to be crystalline-shaped. The same silicon material was used each time. The color and crystalline structure of the deposits varied accor-

[1] Universitätsklinik und Poliklinik für Hals-, Nasen- und Ohrenkranke im Kopfklinikum, D-8700 Würzburg.
[2] Süddeutsches Kunststoffzentrum, D-8700 Würzburg.

Speech Restoration Via Voice Prostheses
Edited by I. F. Herrmann

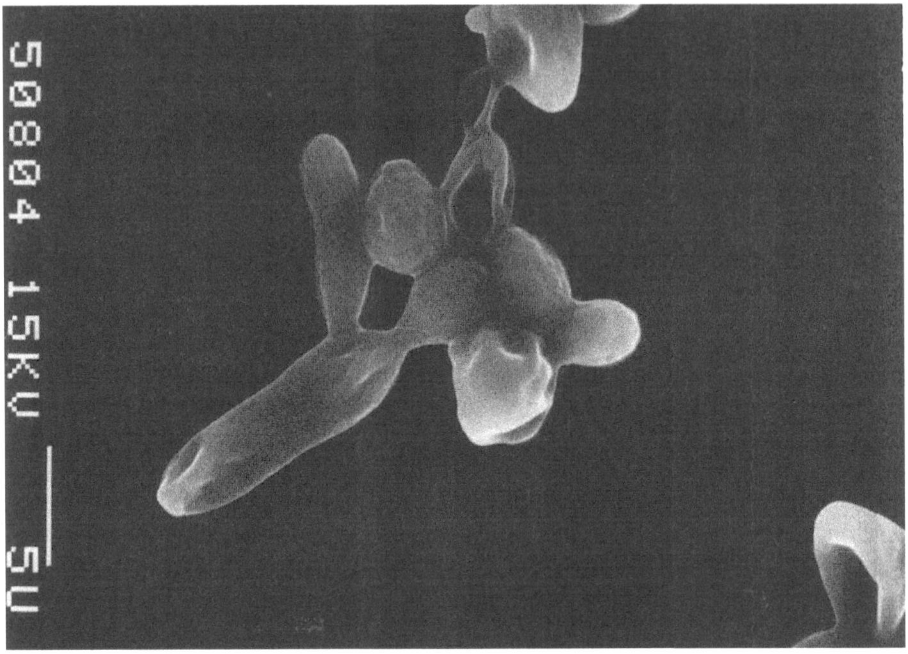

Fig. 1. In vitro colonization of candida albicans on the prosthesis surface. No film can be seen

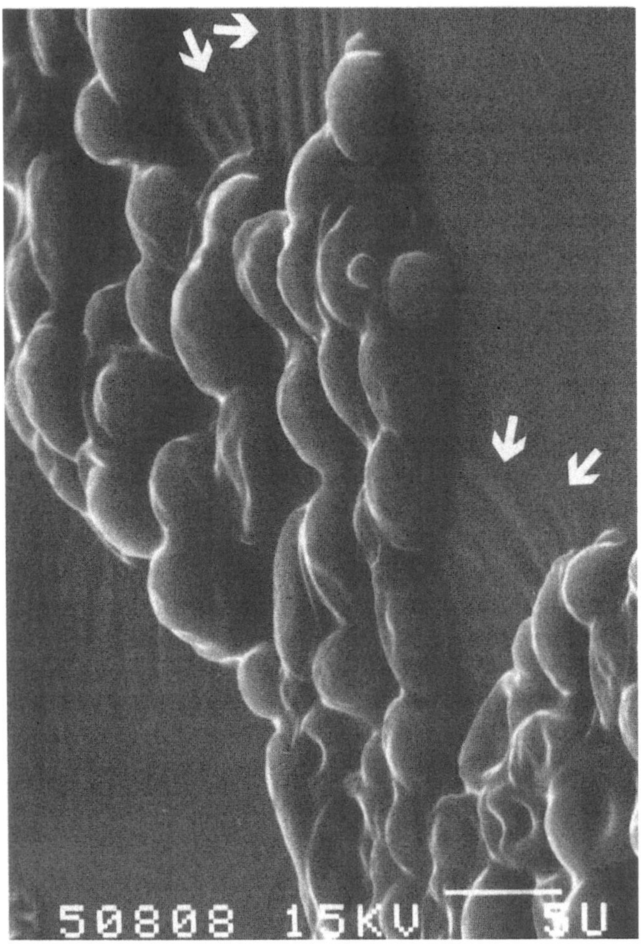

Fig. 2. One day after inserting the prosthesis in the patient a film can be seen on the prosthesis surface (*arrows*). Fungus colonization begins

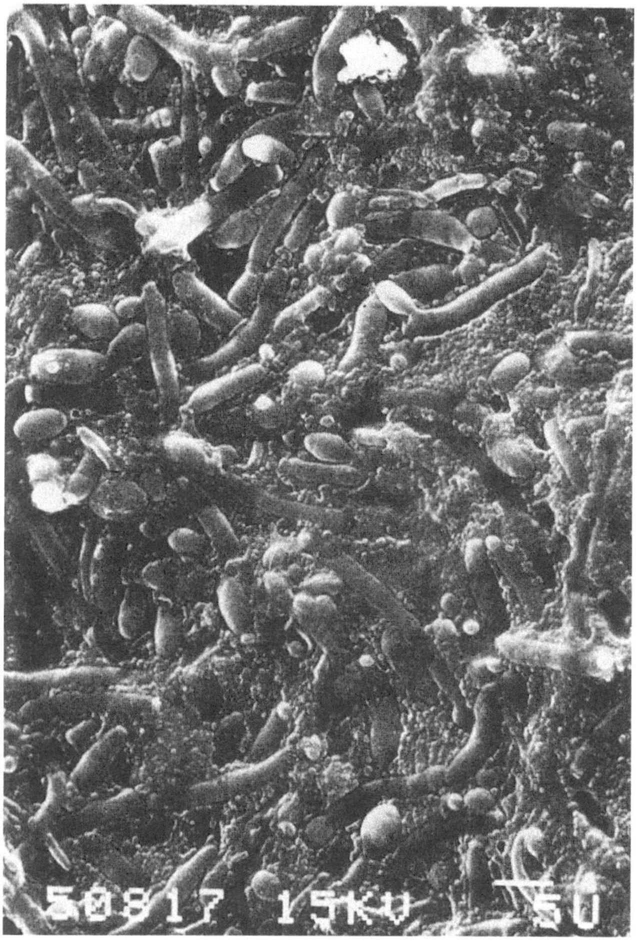

Fig. 3. A little later bacteria and amorphous food particles can be detected in the network of the fungi culture

Fig. 4. Deposits on the surface of a valve lip
▼

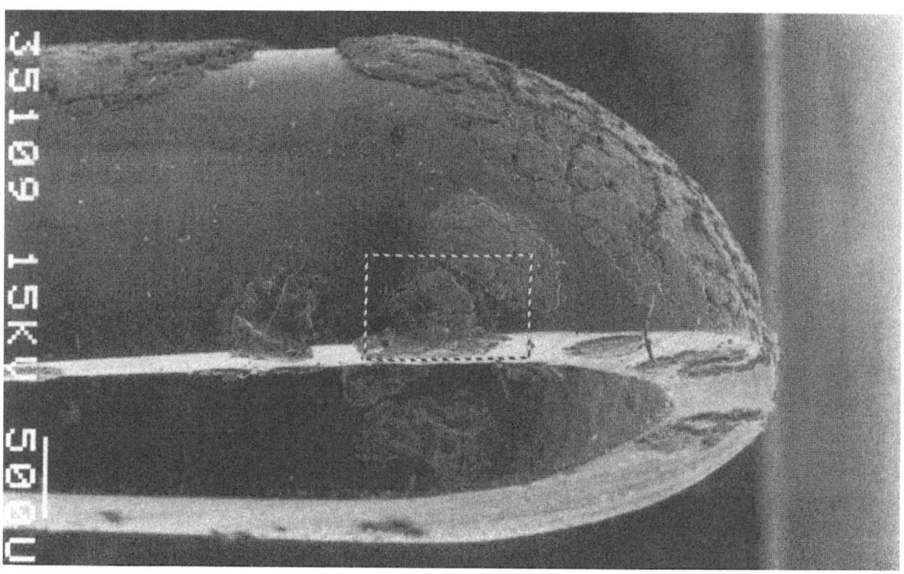

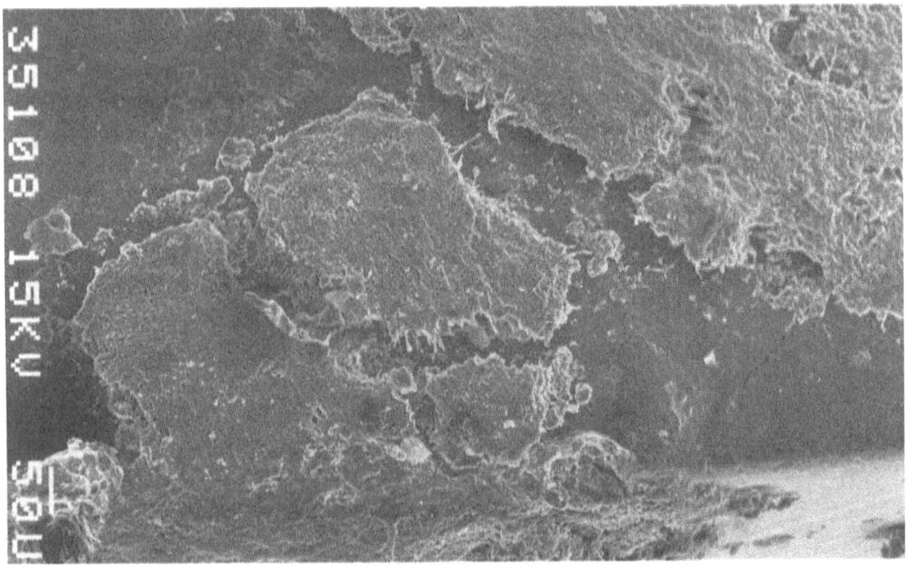

Fig. 5. The same deposits (*broken line* in Fig. 4) using higher magnification

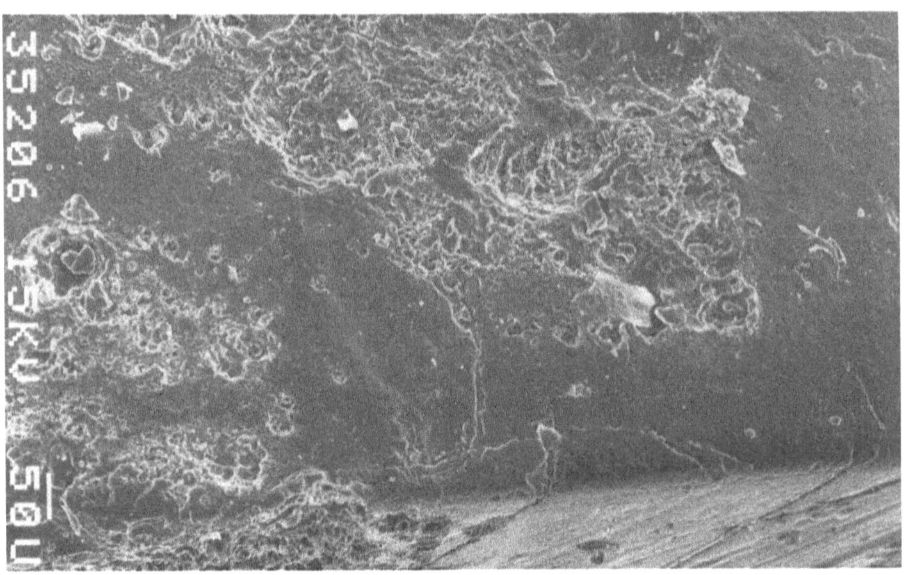

Fig. 6. The deposits have been removed carefully by machine. The change to the silicon material can clearly be seen

ding to the prosthesis user. The deposite were up to 25 μm thick (Fig. 4). It was found that moisture content greatly affects the elasticity of the deposit. Desiccation warped the material and made it brittle. The deposits form mainly in the „voice sphere“ of the valve. Deposits on the sealing surfaces particularly impair proper function (Fig. 5).

The deposits cannot be removed by conventional chemical agents. Nor can they be reduced by 50% and 95% sulphuric acid or 100% acetic acid. Acetic acid increases the volume of the deposit at 50 °C. Sulphuric acid cannot be used at higher temperatures as it would attack the silicon. This is why the deposits are removed carefully by machine when the silicon is being flexed. Figure 6 shows the areas of Fig. 5 once the deposits have been removed. The damage to the silicon material can clearly be seen. It is not known how much is attributable to chemical action.

Analytical (EDX+IR) Investigation

Energy-dispersive X-ray analysis (EDX) as well as electron microscope scanning detect elements whose atomic number is higher than 11, i.e., aluminium. Silicon with traces of calcium, copper, and zinc were mainly found in the valve surface deposits. An infra-red spectroscopic (IR) investigation also indicated the presence of silicates. This points to there being an interaction between the prosthesis material and the ambient media. More detailed experiments are currently being conducted. Any possible effects the material and processes employed may have will be the subject of careful consideration.

Biocompatibility of Plastic Materials

A. SCHAUER [1]

Introduction

The introduction of polymers has brought many exciting developments over the last few decades. The biomedical application of polymers is established in such areas as cardiac and vascular surgery as well as in the application of voice prostheses (Singer and Blom 1980; Henley-Cohn 1981; Herrmann et al. 1983). Many polymers have been and still are in use which have not undergone sufficient preclinical compatibility tests before surgical introduction. According to Ulrich and Bonk (1983) and many other investigators, the most important considerations as to whether polymers are suitable biomedical material are as follows:

Prostheses should contain mostly pure polymers with a minimum of additives and residual catalysts. They should also exhibit the necessary chemical, physical, and mechanical properties for implantation in a living system.

Polymer prostheses should not be adversely affected by the biological environment nor induce any foreign body, inflammatory reaction, encapsulation, or change of the cell response in the surrounding tissue. The polymer should not cause any antileucotactic response or induce tumor formation. Good blood compatibility is essential.

Experience with Biomaterials

In general, tests must be carried out in accordance with the following three stages so as to meet the above criteria:

First stage: A series of preclinical tests and studies in animals and in vitro systems

Second stage: "Use tests" with animals which simulate the human situation

Third stage: Clinical trials on human beings if positive results have been obtained from the above two stages.

As far as silicon voice prostheses are concerned, most of the above criteria have already been met by the implementation of silicon material, e.g., in cardiac valve prostheses or breast inlays. Different compatibility criteria are required for different complexes and such criteria are not always universally relevant. For instance, considerations as to possible thrombogenic properties are especially relevant to vascular prostheses.

[1] Pathologisches Institut der Universität Göttingen, D-3400 Göttingen.

Speech Restoration Via Voice Prostheses
Edited by I. F. Herrmann

Our specific area of research raises the following questions:

1. Is the material resistant enough to body fluids? Or, how soluble is the material?
2. Is the material antigenic per se, or does antigenicity develop after implantation?
3. In what way is the healing process affected in the surrounding area? Is there a special protein adsorption? Is the material angiogenic? Or does the material induce fibroblastic proliferation? How susceptible to infection is the material with regard to protein adsorption?
4. Is there any danger of aspirating silicon particles and the subsequent development of silicon granulomas in the lung?

The following conclusions can be drawn from the current literature:

ad 1. In vitro methods were used to screen possible biomaterials at an early development stage. The test materials were placed in different hydrolytic solutions, e.g., buffer solutions, proteinfluids etc. to determine their solubility.

The degree of solubility was determined by measuring the molecular weights of superficial particles of the polymer before and after implantation. Measurements were made at different time intervals and were substance related. To date, no fundamental or systematic research studies exist on the local conditions of silicon voice prostheses. However, we do know from the use of silicon prostheses in breast surgery that solubility, at least under soft tissue conditions, is very low. As Poschet et al. (1984) pointed out in the workshop, they found severe destruction in the surface layers of voice prostheses after 6 months prosthesis wear. Scanning electron microscopic studies revealed elution of the silicon material. These results are only preliminary and need further systematic investigation.

ad 2. Previous studies, which have investigated antigenicity on the molecular level, have shown that many proteins, synthetic homo- or heteropolypeptides, nucleic acids, as well as homo- and heteropolysaccharides induce antibodies in many animal species. Antibody formation essentially requires a reasonably high molecular weight. The actual nature of the product and the sequence of the composing units are not so important. In other words, a possible immunological response to many of the synthetic polymers currently used as biomaterials cannot be ruled out. Wang (1982) reported that antibodies were produced against sodium polystyrene sulfonate (PSS) and polyacrylacid (PAA) 3–7 days after their implantation in C 57 BL-mice. Antibodies were produced against polyacrylamide (PAM) in SJL-mice. None of these polymers, however, induced humoral antibodies in A, BALB/C, and CBA-mouse strains. This strain-dependent antibody formation clearly shows how the immunological response to synthetic polymers is genetically controlled.

Furthermore, recent information has been gathered on the direct immune response to silicon material. Heggers et al. (1983) tested the biocompatibility of silicon implants and found a 45% inhibition of macrophage migration. Furthermore, a cytoplasmic silicon transfer was found to exist from macrophages to lymphocytes via cytoplasmic bridges.

On the basis of these results, it was concluded that silicon acts as an incomplete hapten-like antigen. As far as we know, however, silicon plays no important

Table 1. Plasmaproteins affecting cellular interactions with foreign materials

Protein	Plasma concentration mg/ml	Material	Celltype	Response
Complement C 3	1.2	Cellophane	Granulocytes	Acute leucopenia
		Mineral oil		Phagocytosis enhanced
		Staph. aureus		Attachment enhanced
Immuno-glob. G	10 –30	Glass	Platelet	Adhesion and release enhanced
		PV-toluene	Granulocytes	Phagocytosis enhanced
			Fibroblasts	Adhesion prevented
Cold insoluble globulin	0.1– 0.3	Falcon dishes	Fibroblasts	Adhesion enhanced
		RE test	Macrophages	Phagocytosis enhanced
		Emulsion	Platelets	
		PVC		Thrombus enhanced
Fibrinogen	3 – 5	Polystyrene	Fibroblasts	Adhesion enhanced
		Silicone rubber	Red blood cells	Adhesion prevented
		Glass		
Albumin	40 –60	Glass	Platelets	Adhesion and release decreased
		Polyethylen	Red cells	Strength of adhesion decreased
		Falcon dishes	Fibroblasts	Adhesion prevented

role in triggering general immune processes after the implantation of a compact prosthesis.

ad 3. Horbett's excellent work (1982) provided new ideas about the interaction problem between the surfaces of polymeric implants and the biological environments concerned. The main point he raises is the existence of a specific or at least highly characteristic interaction between the components of the adsorbed protein layer and the peripheral cells. Such observations led to the hypothesis that local reactions around the polymer are controlled by the presence of a specific protein coating sufficiently dense on one side and with sufficient reactive cellular potential to elicit a response on the other side. Of the plasma proteins probably only those with specific cellular receptors, for instance fibrinogen or platelet proteins, can strengthen the intensive and specific responses of a special cell type. Other proteins such as albumins inhibit rather than elicit cellular reactions in certain cases (Table 1).

Horbett's experiments (1982) demonstrate clearly that the specific balance between "reactive" and "non-reactive" proteins is determined by biomaterial surface chemistry which is the result of affinity differences among the proteins. In contrast to these interactions, the polymer material may induce only slight or nonactive cellular response. They become indirectly reactive by selecting and interfacially concentrating specific proteins from the bulk phase to the surface phase.

It can be concluded that the characteristic composition of the adsorbed protein layer and the reactivity of the protein molecules within this layer may affect the local cellular response specifically.

Our experiment with a silicon prosthesis showed that silicon rubber and silicon glass lead to the adsorption of fibrinogen in particular and enhance fibroblastic activity.

Two serious factors require further consideration:

1. The fibrinogen adsorption of the polymer serves as a good "depot" for bacterial infection.
2. From a theoretical point of view, an abundant fibrillation together with the facultative development of fibroid pseudopolyps takes place which may be responsible for the partial obstruction of the respiratory pathway.

There are no indications to suggest that special additional angioformative factors might play any important role (Fig. 1). In our opinion, polymer material interactions affecting the local milieu require further and extensive morphological, physical and microbiological evaluation by the most modern techniques of all the disciplines concerned.

Scanning electron microscopy shows that silicon material-surfaces are not very smooth and reveals squamous-like pictures. The use of metallic material such as gold vapour, to improve the surface layers did not produce satisfactory results.

ad 4. Cardiac surgery has provided us with some knowledge about silicongranuloma formation. When low quality silicon balls were first used, silicon material was desquamated and silicon microembolies developed in different organs, especially in the kidney and in the liver. This process introduced thousands of foreign body granulomas into these organs. The same occurs when silicon-dust is inhaled. Intensive granuloma formation develops in lung parenchyma. One cannot assume that the same will happen when using and changing the voice prosthesis. However, it cannot be ruled out that surface particles might reach the lung and develop single or multiple granulomas.

ad 5. Polymer-carcinogenesis is a pathogenetically unclear process and has been discussed for a long time. The discussion began in the late 1950s when different laboratories detected sarcomas after polymers had been implanted in the soft tissue of different animal species.

The work of Bischoff et al. (1972) and also of Brand et al. (1980) provides further information about this problem. In collections of single cases of human fore-

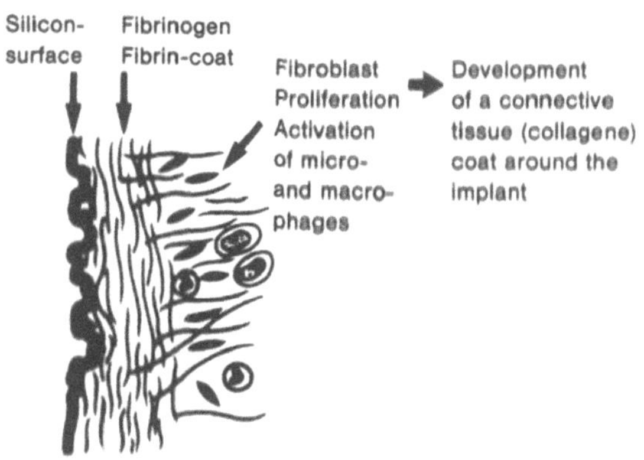

Fig. 1. Reactions around silicon implants

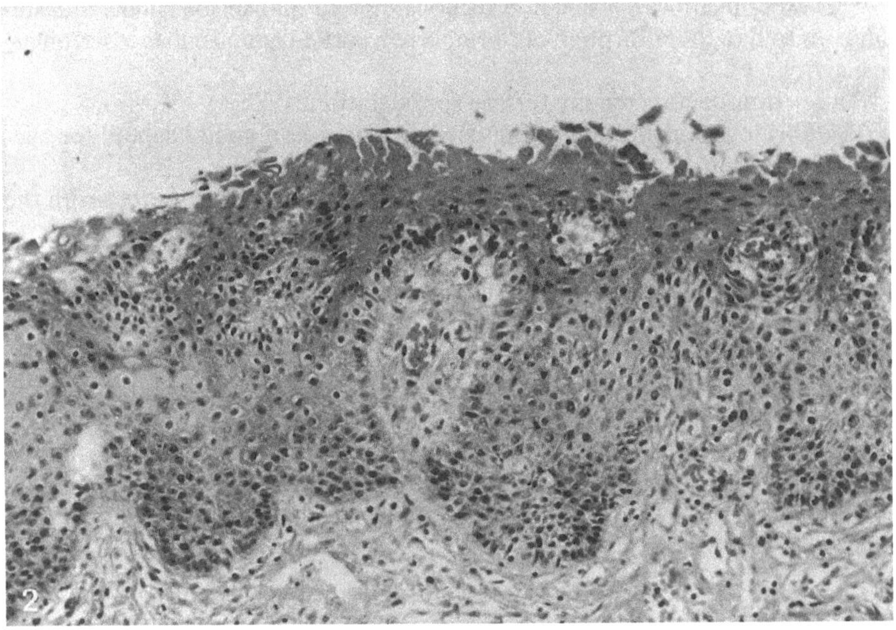

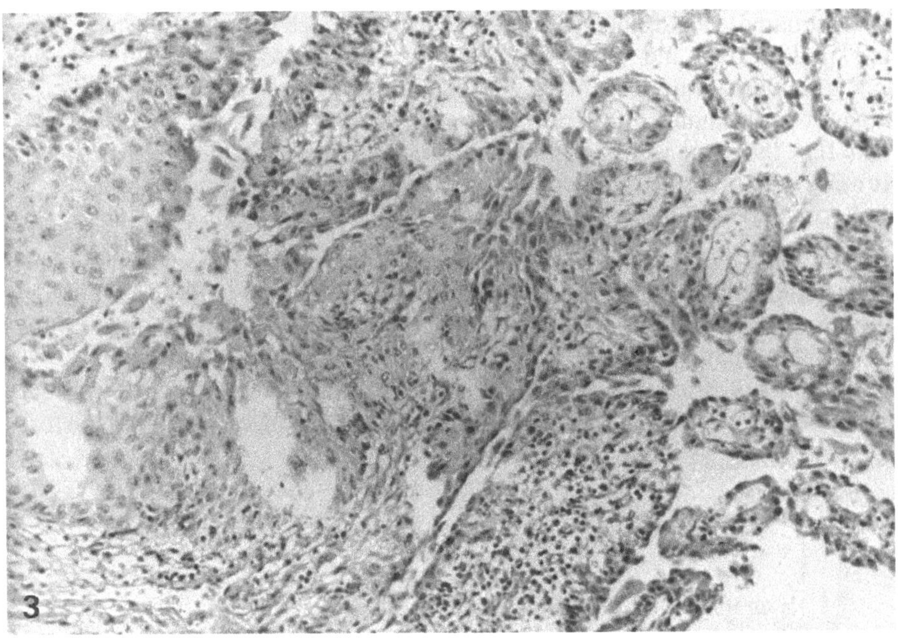

Fig. 2. Squamous metaplasia of the respiratory mucosa with low grade dysplasia near the prosthesis: chronic inflammation. No atypical changes. HE-stain

Fig. 3. Squamous metaplasia with papillary hyperplasia and chronic inflammatory reaction near the prosthesis. No atypia of the epithelium. HE-stain

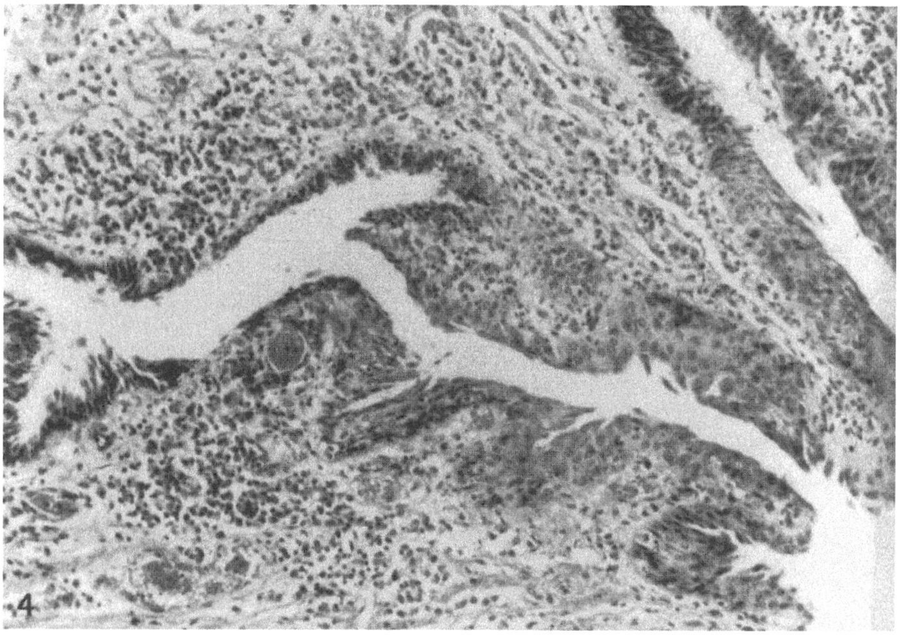

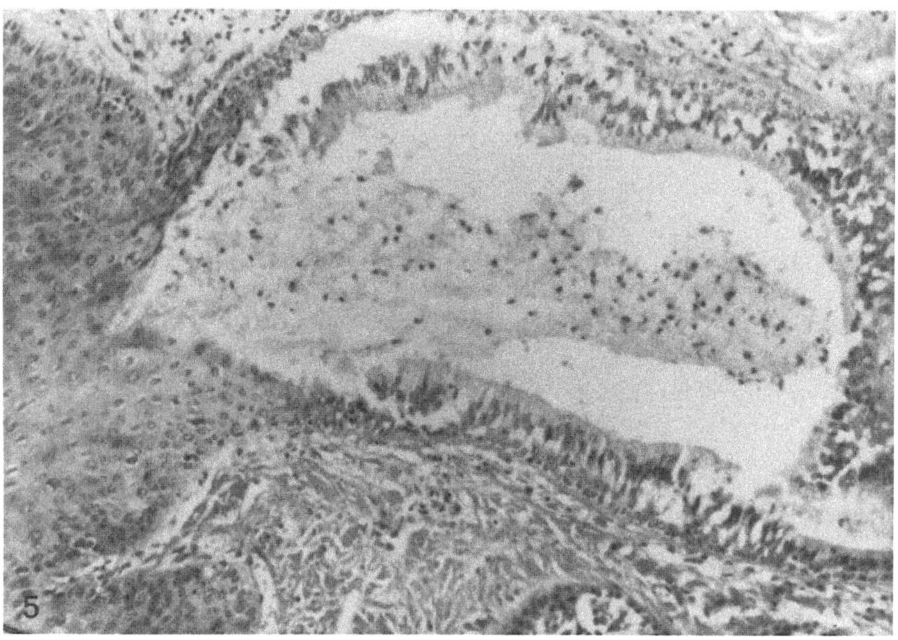

Fig. 4. Papillary proliferation of the surface epithelium also with squamous metaplasia of the superficial parts of glandular duct epithelium. Severe chronic inflammatory reaction of the local stroma. HE-stain

Fig. 5. Squamous metaplasia of the surface epithelium. Ballooning of mucous gland ducts following duct occlusion. HE-stain

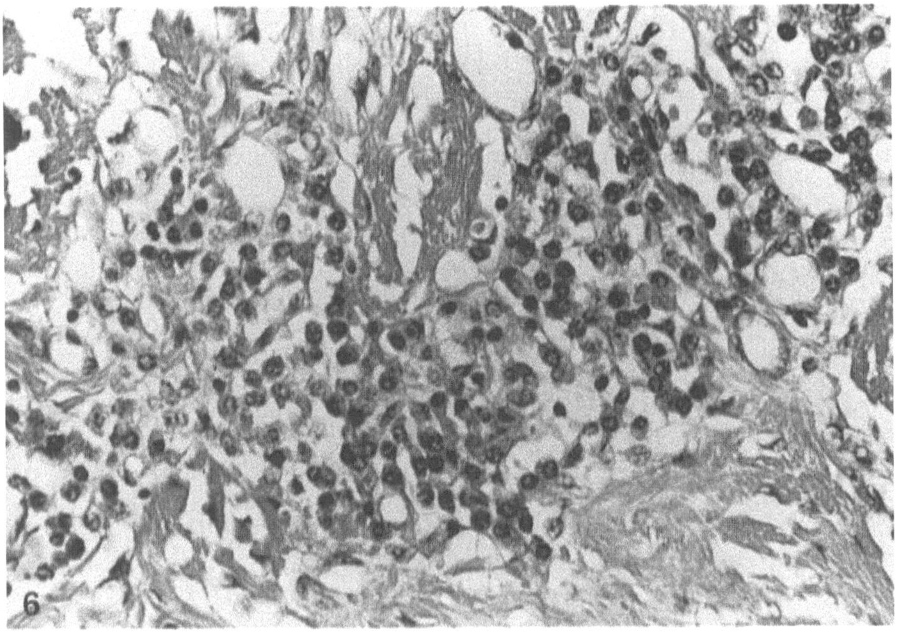

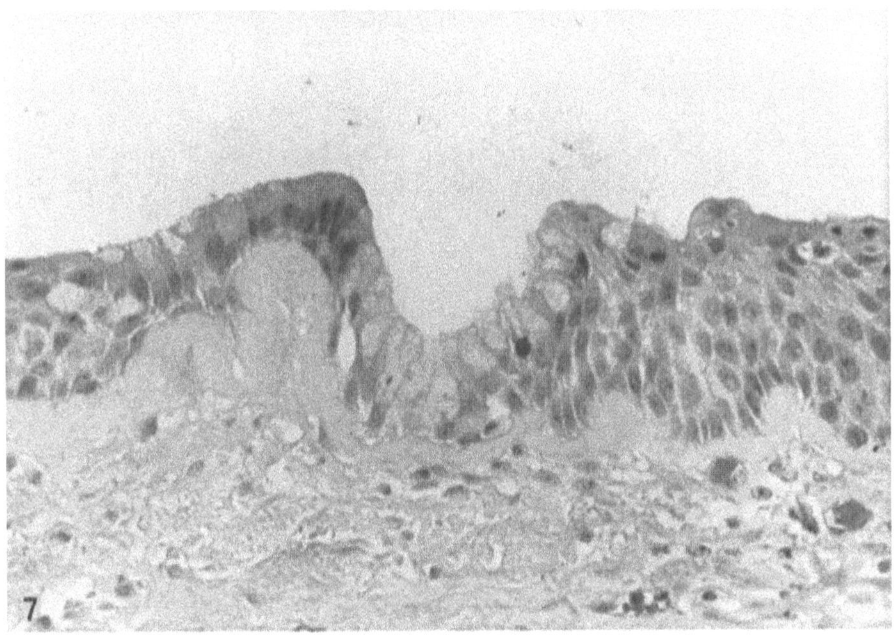

Fig. 6. Severe chronic inflammatory reaction with lymphocytes and plasma cells in the submucosal stroma near the voice prosthesis. HE-stain

Fig. 7. Beginning squamous metaplasia of the surface epithelium (*right*), respiratory epithelium with goblet cells in the *middle* part of the picture (baboon). Some weeks after implantation of the voice prosthesis. HE-stain

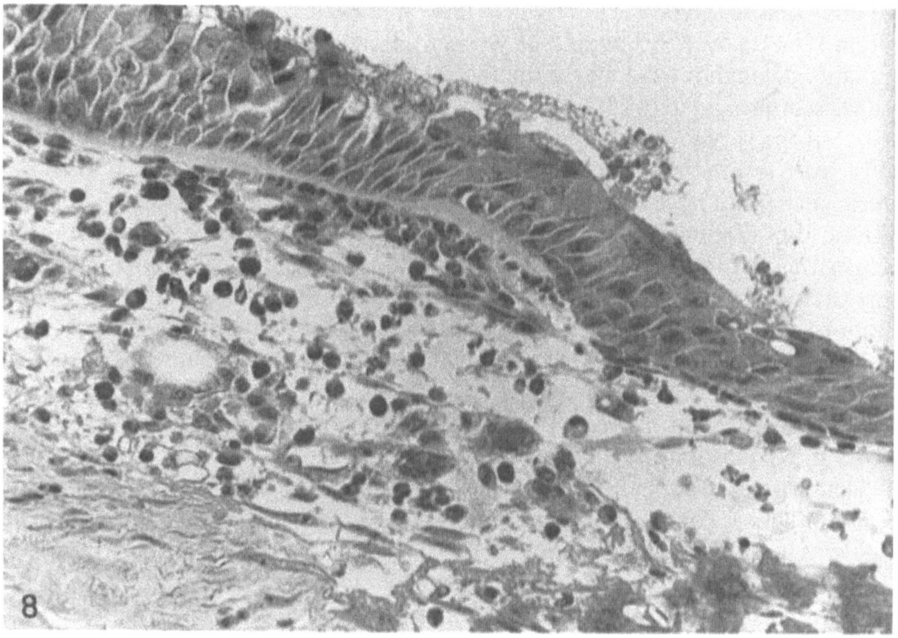

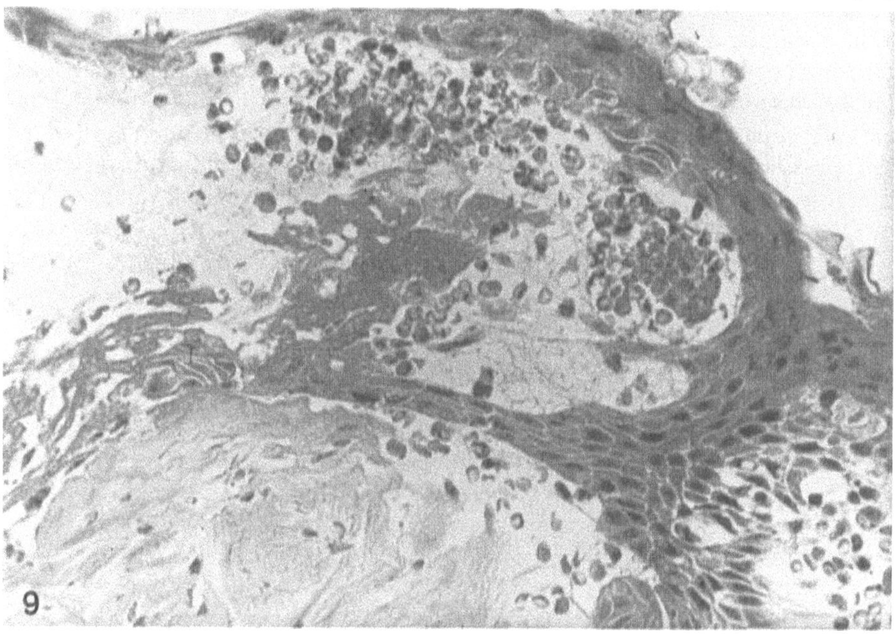

Fig. 8. Squamous metaplasia of the respiratory epithelium around the voice prosthesis some weeks after implantation (baboon). Subepithelial edema and inflammatory reaction. HE-stain

Fig. 9. Squamous metaplasia of the respiratory epithelium near the voice prosthesis. Severe subepithelial edema with inflammatory reaction some weeks after implantation (baboon). HE-stain ign body and scar related cancers with known latencies, over 25% had developed within 15 years over 50% within 25 years. Millions of patients have been carrying implants throughout the world for the past 10–20 years. According to this hypothesis, approximately 25% of these patients ought to have developed cancer by now, but the very low occurrence rate observed hitherto indicates that incidence will remain low in the future. Brand et al. (1980) developed a test system to detect precancer cells in mice after the implantation of foreign body material. This test showed that precancer cells can be found at high levels before the development of invasive sarcomas. 27 human tissue specimens were taken from implant regions only to find a negative precancer cell result. The results of these and other investigations show that implant-induced cancers in man are rare but do exist.

Therefore, it is necessary to test implant materials as to their degree of carcinogenicity before implantation. Further technical, biochemical, immunological, and microbiological investigations with morphological methods are needed to clarify these questions.

Histological examinations in the voice prosthesis region: Our own morphological, microbiological, and immunological research of the above-mentioned problems is still incomplete.

Figures 2–6 show the local changes and reactions which occurred around the ostium of the voice prosthesis of a 56 year old patient, who died from cardiac failure about four years after implantation. Partial papillary squamous metaplasia of the glandular ducts which balloon after occlusion near the metaplastic surface epithelium as well as chronic inflammatory reactions are the most striking local changes observed by routine morphological methods. Furthermore, Figs. 7–9 reveal early squamous metaplastic changes of the respiratory epithelium around the voice prosthesis of a baboon a few weeks after implantation. Submucosal edema and severe inflammatory reaction were found in the submucosal layers.

Summary

One of the major problems after the implantation of a silicon voice prosthesis is that of local infection. This problem may be at least partly connected with polymer fibrinogen and other protein interactions. Another serious problem is the stimulation of fibroblastic and local mesenchymal activity in the prosthesis contact region with the intensive fibroblastic proliferation or formation of so-called fibroid polyps. In comparison with these factors, all the other aspects discussed in this paper are of minor significance for long-term implant compatibility.

References

Bischoff F (1972) Organic polymer biocompatibility and toxicology (Review). Clinical Chemistry 18:869

Blom ED, Singer MJ, Hamaker RC (1982) Tracheostoma valve for postlaryngectomy voice rehabilitation. Ann Otol 91:576

Brand KG, Brand I (1980) Risk assessment of carcinogenesis at implantation sites. Surgery 66:591

Heggers JP et al. (1983) Biocompatibility of silicone implants. Ann Plast Surg 11:38–45

Henley-Cohn J (1981) How I do it – head and neck. A targeted problem and its solution. New technique for insertion of laryngeal prosthesis. Laryngoscope 91:1957

Herrmann IF, Zenner HP (1984) Erfahrungen mit der Blom-Singer-Prothese nach Blom-Singer-Punktion und nach funktionsgestörter Neoglottis phonatoria. HNO 32:286–293

Horbett TA (1982) Protein adsorption on biomaterials. Biomaterials: Interfacial phenomena and applications. Advances in chemistry series. American Chemical Society, Washington D.C.

Karschay P et al. (1986) Untersuchungen zur chirurgischen Stimmrehabilitation bei Verwendung von Ventilprothesen. Acta Otolaryngica 101:341–347

Poschet G et al. (1984) Wearing of silicon during exposition of valve prosthesis in the upper digestive tract – a study using scanning electron microscopy. International workshop on voice prosthesis strategies for speech restoration, Würzburg

Singer MI, Blom ED (1980) An endoscopic technique for restoration of voice after laryngectomy. Ann Otol 89:529

Ulrich H, Bonk HW (1983) Emerging biomedical applications of polyurethan elastomers. Reprinted from the meeting of the minds. Marketing of the SPI 27th annual meeting technical marketing conference

Wang PY (1982) On the antigenicity of synthetic biomedical polymers. In: Winter JD et al. (eds) Biomaterials 1980.

Chapter 3 In Vivo Experiments Using Voice Prostheses

Aerodynamic Properties of Buttons and Button-Assisted Oesophageal Speech

G. L. J. Nieboer and H. K. Schutte[1]

Introduction

The last three years have produced several articles on button aerodynamics. Weinberg, Horii, and Singer and Blom (Weinberg et al. 1982; Weinberg 1982) have described experimental settings to measure the airflow resistance of the Blom-Singer and Panje buttons. In the Groningen ENT Clinic, we have made comparative measurements with four types of buttons. We have also made pressure and flow measurements on button speakers.

In Vitro Measurements of Buttons: Pressure, Flow and Resistance

The four button types we used are shown in Fig. 1. The Groningen and the Blom-Singer button were further developed after we made our measurements.

For aerodynamic measurements, it is convenient to divide the buttons into a tube part and a valve part. This division can be seen in Fig. 1 where the tube parts

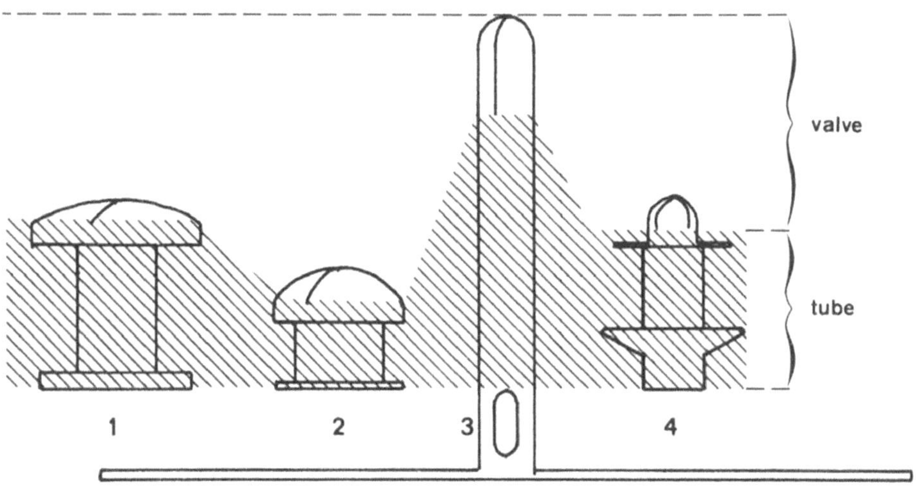

Fig. 1. The 4 button types we tested. *1*, Groningen button, *2*, Groningen Staffieri button (for patients with neoglottis according to Staffieri), *3*, Blom-Singer button (old model), *4*, Panje button. The tube parts have been shaded

[1] ENT Clinic Academic Hospital Groningen, 9700 RB Groningen, The Netherlands.

Speech Restoration Via Voice Prostheses
Edited by I. F. Herrmann

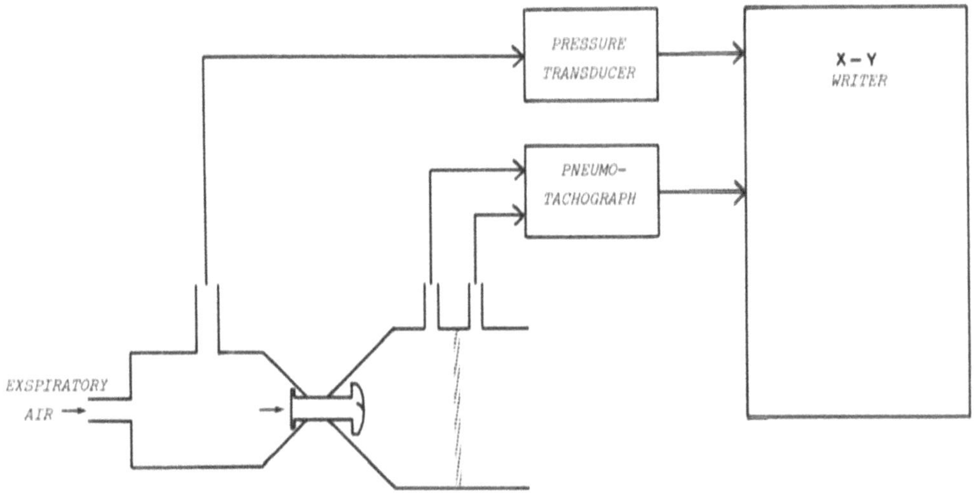

Fig. 2. Experimental setting for button testing

have been shadowed. Figure 2 shows the experimental setting used in our measurements. The button is placed in a small device which enables the researcher to measure the air pressure at the inlet and outlet of the button. In order to simulate the in vivo situation, normal expiratory air is used in these experiments. The buttons are allowed to warm up before the actual measurements are taken.

The outcome of each test is expressed as an X-Y graph showing the pressure/flow relationship (Fig. 3). Two things can be read from such graphs. Firstly, button resistance can be computed by dividing the pressure (in kPa) by the flow (in l/s). We chose air flow values of 0.025, 0.05, 0.15, 0.25, and 0.35 l/s, which cover the whole range of flow values found for our in vivo measurements during oesophageal speech.

Secondly, these graphs give information on the opening pressure, i.e., the amount of pressure needed to open the valve. It is clear that the button valve must be completely closed when no pressure is exerted on either valve side. So as to avoid leakage, the opening pressure can be measured by observing the point on the graph where the straight line, indicating zero flow, begins to move to the right. The opening pressures we recorded (Table 1) are based on a small number of measurements. Their only worth is to show that opening pressure is an important parameter for aerodynamic testing. Opening pressure should not be too high. The same applies for button airflow resistance. This resistance should be as low as possible in order to obtain the highest possible flow and subglottic pressure. The oesophageal voice mechanism will then function in the most efficient way. Physiological problems will also be avoided which arise from the very high intratracheal pressures. When we plot the resistance values of the buttons on a graph, however, they can be somewhat misleading (Fig. 4). When there is a certain amount of pressure, e.g., when the valve is closed and there is no flow, the resistance will be infinitely high. Therefore, it is better to work in terms of pressure loss or pressure drop over the button rather than in terms of resistance.

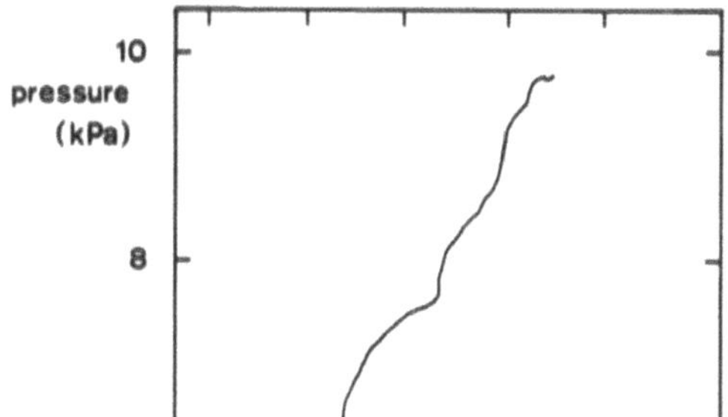

Fig. 3. X-Y graph of the pressure/flow relationship found after testing one button. Both the opening pressure and airflow resistance can be read from this graph

However, there is at least some information which these resistance values can give us. Firstly, high resistance to low flow values indicates good valve closure. On the other hand, high resistance to high flow values means that the tube part, or the valve opening, are rather small. In this case, resistance will increase, at least with laminar flow, because it depends on the radius or opening of the tube to the 4th power. This brings us to the resistance of the tube parts of the buttons (Table 2). We simulated buttons without valves: for these measurements the air was blow through smooth-walled tubes of the same size as the tube parts of the buttons (see Fig. 1). The part played by the pressure drop of the button during conversation must not be neglected. During the loudest phonation, the Panje and old Blom-Singer model button tubes are responsible for a maximum of 23% and 17% of the overall button pressure drop, respectively.

Table 1. Opening pressure in kPa of the button valve parts

Blom-Singer button	0.0
Panje button	0.0
Groningen button	0.5
Groningen-Staffieri button	0.2

Table 2. Percentage of button tube part resistance for the flow values of 0.15 and 0.35 l/s

	0.15 l/s	0.35 l/s
Groningen button	2%	3%
Groningen-Staffieri button	1%	1.5%
Blom-Singer button	14%	17%
Panje button	15%	23%

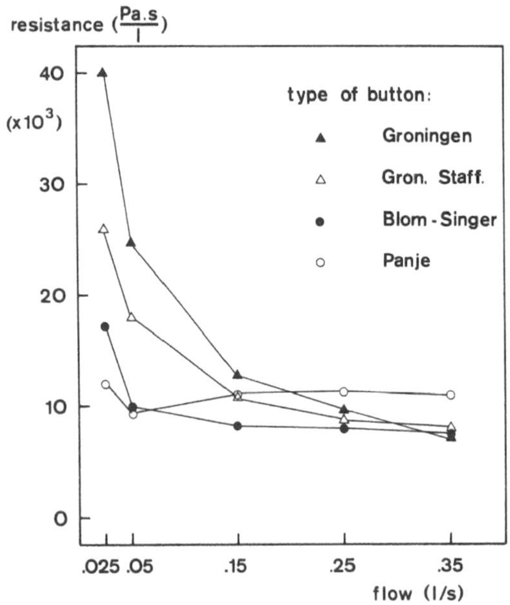

Fig. 4. Resistance of the 4 button types to 5 different air flow rates

In Vivo Measurements: Airflow, Pressure, and Intensity

In 7 Groningen button patients, we measured simultaneously the intratracheal pressure, the oral/nasal flow, and the sound intensity of a large number of phonations. We also measured the intraoesophageal pressure of a few patients with an oesophageal balloon. These measurements revealed that only the supraclavicular part of the oesophagus takes part in the phonation of oesophageal button speakers. We recorded very high intratracheal pressures. During loud phonation, some patients reached a pressure of up to 12 kPa. During comfortable phonation, a pressure of 3 to 5 kPa was applied.

One can easily calculate the intraoesophageal pressure from this intratracheal pressure by subtracting the button pressure drop from the latter. We found that this button pressure drop during button-assisted phonation was up to 20% in conversational voice (Table 3), with flow values of 0.1–0.15 l/s. When we compared these data with those of Weinberg and others (Weinberg et al. 1982; Weinberg 1982), we noted that these researchers found higher resistance values for the buttons. In speakers using a Panje type button, the prosthesis accounted for up to 60% of the driving pressure in the trachea. We suggest that our data are different due to the different air composition and temperature we used in our measurements. Weinberg used air from a cylinder which was probably normal air. We used expiratory air and allowed the buttons to become both wet and warm before we took any measurements so as to simulate an in vivo situation. In fact, we did find higher resistance values in buttons which had not been allowed to warm up. Moreover, the differences shown in Fig. 3 would have been even greater if Weinberg had taken the resistance of the tube parts of the button into account.

Table 3. The approximate percentages of the pressure losses (equal to the intratracheal pressure minus the intraoesophageal pressure) in three button types calculated by the authors and by Weinberg (Weinberg et al. 1982; Weinberg, 1982)

		Weinberg
Groningen button	c. 20%	
Panje button	c. 20%	c. 60%
Blom-Singer button	c. 15%	c. 30%

Conclusions

Our first conclusion from these investigations is that all 4 of the button types we tested, are only responsible for a small part of high intratracheal pressures. This does not exclude, of course, other factors which can influence button resistance, e.g., oeosphageal tissue contact or aging of the silicon material. Secondly, we have drawn a tentative conclusion that the oesophagus must be considered a passive air container during button-assisted oesophageal phonation. The driving force originates from the expiratory mechanism. In fact, this will be one of the objects of investigation in a 3-year research program on button-assisted oesophageal speech in the Groningen ENT Clinic. Thirdly, we may conclude that Groningen buttons have a low tube part resistance and a functional valve mechanism.

References

Nijdam HF, Annyas AA, Schutte HK, Leever H (1982) A new prosthesis for voice rehabilitation after laryngectomy. Arch Otorhinolaryngol 237:27–33

Weinberg B (1982) Airway resistance of the voice button. Arch Otolaryngol 108:498–500

Weinberg B, Horii Y, Blom E, Singer M (1982) Airway resistance during esophageal phonation. J Speech Hear Disord 47:194–199

In Vivo Experiments Using Valve Prostheses – Resistance and Pressure/Time Measurement

S. WALTER, U. KNÖLLINGER and I. F. HERRMANN [1]

Methods

Airway resistance during phonation and the influence of valve prosthesis and radiotherapy on aerodynamics are major points of interest. We have therefore taken resistance and pressure/time measurements.

First we measured the airway resistance characteristics of the Blom-Singer-prosthesis and the ESKA-Herrmann prosthesis. Then we took the measurements of alaryngeal speakers during phonation. Air flow was measured by a baby-pneumotachograph and by a differential pressure transducer. Air pressure was recorded by a pressure transducer. The results of the measurements were shown on a channel-recorder.

1. Aerodynamics of the Valve Prostheses

The aerodynamics of the prostheses are characterized by the airway resistance R which is derived from the ratio between transdevice pressure and transdevice flow:

$$R = \Delta P / \Delta Q.$$

The relationship between pressure and flow is mostly linear within the expected phonatory flow range up to 150 ml/s. Airway resistance therefore remains relatively constant and the following values were found:

Blom-Singer Prosthesis $R = 10$ Pa/ml/s
ESKA-Herrmann Prosthesis $R = 16$ Pa/ml/s

2. Aerodynamics of Alaryngeal Speakers

We used the same pneumotachograph and pressure transducers mentioned above for measuring our patients.

The patient wore an anaesthetic mask connected to the pneumotachograph when the air flow was recorded. Air pressure was recorded by closing the tracheostoma cannula with a small tube connected to the pressure transducer. Each patient was asked to produce a sustained "a" sound and to reduce loudness until loss of speech. Air flow and air pressure were then recorded simultaneously.

In order to compare several different surgical methods, we used the constant differential airway resistance $R = \Delta P / \Delta Q$ and the critical pressure P_k which is necessary for minimal phonation and created by the pharyngeal muscles.

[1] Universitätsklinik und Poliklinik für Hals-, Nasen- und Ohrenkranke im Kopfklinikum, D-8700 Würzburg.

Speech Restoration Via Voice Prostheses
Edited by I. F. Herrmann

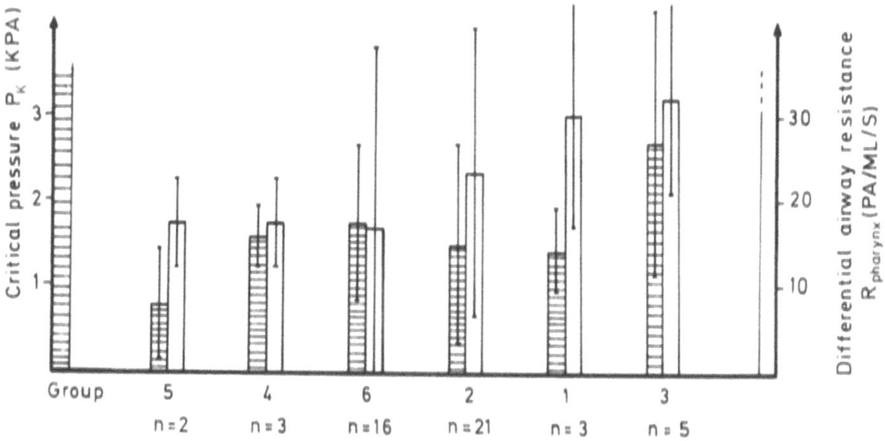

Fig. 1. Mean and standard deviation ($\bar{x} \pm s$) of airway resistance R and critical pressure P_k

a) Comparison of Several Surgical Techniques

All the patients taking part in the comparison were provided with an "ESKA-Herrmann Prosthesis". They were then divided into groups according to the surgical technique employed during their operation:

Group 1: puncture method
Group 2: glottoplasty type I and II
Group 3: glottoplasty type I and II; partial pharyngectomy without reconstruction of pharynx
Group 4: glottoplasty type I and II; partial pharyngectomy with additional reconstruction of pharynx
Group 5: glottoplasty type III
Group 6: glottoplasty with functional pharynx surgery and tracheostomaplasty

The average results obtained are given in Fig. 1. The differential resistance R is described as airway resistance $R_{pharynx}$, which is caused by anatomical structures. It represents the results obtained minus the resistance of the prosthesis.

A comparison of the surgical groups reveals how the reconstruction of the pharynx after a partial pharyngectomy is the cause of an enormous reduction in resistance and pressure during phonation (Groups 3 and 4).

The aerodynamic data of glottoplasty (Groups 2, 4, 5, 6) are approximately one third less than those obtained by puncture methods (Group 1). Glottoplasty (i.e., the construction of a tracheo-oesophageal shunt in one stage with the laryngectomy) seems to provide better aerodynamic results than with a puncture.

b) Comparison of Several Prostheses

A comparison of the Blom-Singer and the ESKA-Herrmann prostheses reveals that the latter creates about half as much pressure and resistance as the former. One patient was able to be measured with both prostheses after using the Blom-Singer technique and the hypopharyngeal puncture technique. Obvious differences are caused by the prostheses and their correct position.

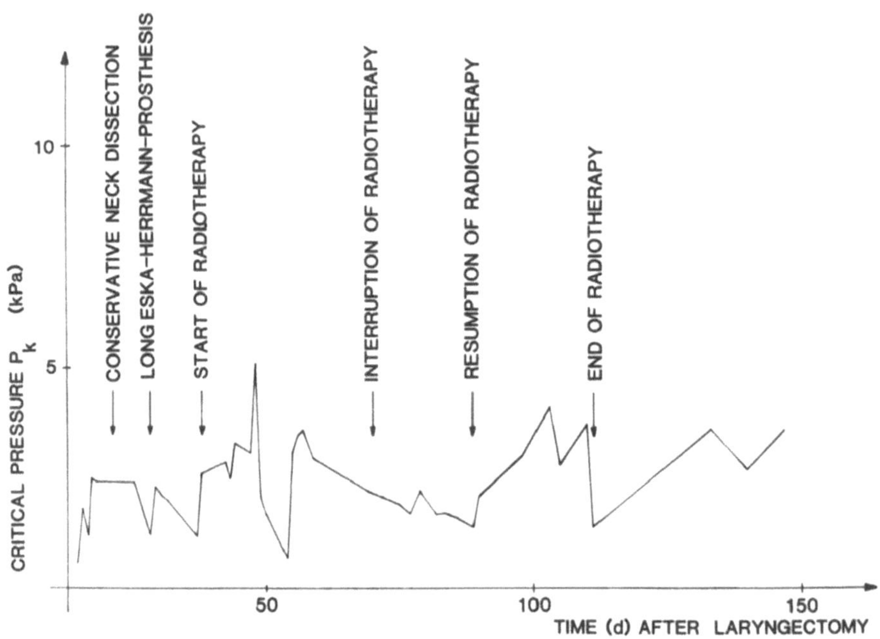

Fig. 2. Postoperative development of critical pressure P_k

The reason for the better results of the ESKA-Herrmann prosthesis in situ can be seen in its flexion which enables the resistant airway of the pharyngeal muscle tube to be shortened.

c) Pressure/Time Measurements and Observation of Postoperative Development

For pressure/time measurements, patients were asked to phonate a certain polysyllable at a comfortable loudness. Air pressure was recorded on the abcissa and time on the ordinate. We calculated the middle pressure of phonation P_s from the resultant curve.

The postoperative development of critical pressure P_k and middle phonation pressure P_s was observed in patients belonging to Group 6 (glottoplasty with functional pharynx surgery). At first, measurements were taken every day immediately after prosthesis insertion (ESKA-Herrmann in all cases) and then at longer intervals (Fig. 2). We compared patients both with and without additional pharynx reconstruction regarding P_k and P_s We found that the negative effects of radiotherapy on phonation (edema, tumefaction, cicatrizing) were clearly less in patients who had undergone additional pharynx reconstruction.

Conclusion

Our in vivo experiments substantiate two presuppositions:

1. The ESKA-Herrmann Prosthesis reduces airway resistance.
2. Additional pharynx reconstruction after partial pharyngectomy reduces the negative affects of radiotherapy on phonation.

Chapter 4 Problems Occurring with the Inferior Pharyngeal Muscle and Their Possible Solutions

Function of the Pharynx and Killian Mouth in Voice Production with Our Prosthesis

L. TRAISSAC, J. PETIT, M. LECOQ, F. DEVARS, M. BENKIRANE, J. Y. NIZOU and F. MOUROT [1]

Introduction

We tried to understand the mechanics of voice production. Since the prosthesis does not have any vibrating structure and is placed under the Killian mouth, its role in voice production appears to be nonexistent with the obvious exception that it allows the passage of air. Thus, we tried to understand the function of the Killian mouth and the pharynx.

Materials and Methods

We made the following different types of studies:

1. A fibroscopic examination to visualize directly the pharynx and Killian mouth during vocalization (and not only for the sounding of a single vowel).
2. An additional stroboscopic examination allowing us to see neoglottis vibrations.
3. An X-ray examination with a brilliance amplifier permitting the analysis of movements of the pharynx, Killian mouth, and prosthesis during voice production.
4. Manometry was also performed at tracheostoma level together with flow measurements at oral cavity level.

A study was carried out with 8 patients who were asked to "hold" an "a", count up to 5, read the same sentence.

The Role of the Killian Mouth (Fig. 1)

1. Its Primary Role as a Sphincter

a) The "cricopharyngeus" is the muscle which forms the Killian mouth. This muscle, severed during the operation, is always stitched to the reconstructed pharyngeal tunnel. It is as if it has becomes hypertrophic and the result is a real sphincter with a circular muscle fold. We can easily visualize this circular muscle fold by means of fibroscopy. It only opens during deglutition when the prosthesis, normally hidden under the crico-oesophageal muscle, can be briefly seen. X-rays

[1] 89 Rue des Sablières, F-33077 Bordeaux Cedex.

Speech Restoration Via Voice Prostheses
Edited by I. F. Herrmann

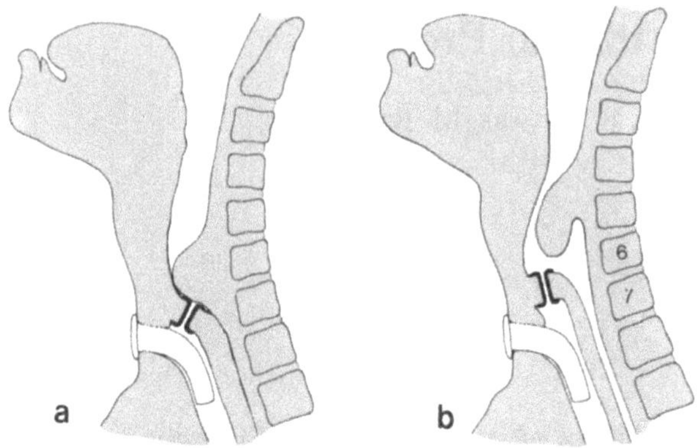

Fig. 1. Position of the Killian mouth and pharynx at rest (*left*) and during phonation of the vowel "a". Drawings from X-rays

reveal it with or without voice production. (N.B. All the patients observed had been wearing the prosthesis for several months. We think that training may play a role in the formation of this muscle fold.)

b) Fibroscopy and radiography with a brilliance amplifier show the kinetics of the Killian mouth. Fibroscopy, often impaired by salivary stasis, shows that voice production occurs after the Killian mouth has contracted. Its contraction begins with a downward movement and leads to a small salivary regurgitation. Voice production, however, begins with an upward movement.

The study of pressures and flows confirms that the Killian mouth works like a sphincter. Our research till now has shown, that voice production only starts when a pressure of 25–30 cm of H_2O has been obtained.

The neoglottis (Killian mouth) is formed solely by the cricopharyngeal muscle whose contraction is less quantifiable than that of the laryngeal muscle. However, it can still be controlled fairly accurately. We noticed that one of our patients had flow increases during vocalization corresponding to a stabilized intratracheal pressure. This implies a controlled relaxation of the superior oesophageal sphincter.

Kinetic studies with a brilliance amplifier also show great mobility of the sphincter during voice production. However, we have not been able to analyze the results with any great accuracy. Therefore, we have not been able to establish a relation between the shape, thickness, or height of this fold and the phoneme emitted. Moreover, these movements are partly passive and are supported by the pharyngeal walls and the base of the tongue.

2. Where Can Vibration Be Seen?

Mucous vibration occurs at the neoglottis level. Stroboscopy performed during fibroscopy reveals the undulating movement of the neoglottis mucous membrane. This undulation is regular and directed upwards. It starts at the same time the neoglottis begins to move. We think that this wave starts at the lower border of the neoglottis and rises towards the upper one.

We tried to establish a correlation between the basic sound emitted and the oesophageal sphincter position. We therefore anaylzed X-rays of the larynx during voice production. It proved impossible to correlate the position, height, or thickness of the oesophageal sphincter with the prosthesis and sound frequency.

It must also be noted that the "bubbly" timbre of the voice obtained is due to salivary stasis above the sphincter during vocalization. It is also important to note that these patients have often already undergone radiotherapy and have bad quality saliva which sticks to the walls.

The Role of The Pharynx

It is more difficult to establish the role of the pharynx.

a) The pharynx does not play any part in voice production. Fibroscopy together with stroboscopy have never revealed vibrations at the pharyngeal wall.

b) We can best visualize the overall kinetics of the pharynx and lower part of the tongue with a brilliance amplifier. We tried to compare the pharynx mobility of patients who had undergone a total laryngectomy with good oesophageal speakers and patients wearing our prosthesis. Among the latter group, the mobility of the pharynx is always much more important. This can be explained by the fact that the ascending air flow does not need injection. It is more important and lasts longer. Its pressure is adaptable and the body diagramme is less disturbed. The pharynx can therefore modulate the voice.

During voice production, the base of the tongue moves as quickly as the tongue itself. It constantly changes the volume of the pharyngeal cavity and determines timbre quality. However, it does not affect sound frequency as this can only be changed by the vibratory zone of the Killian mouth.

Comments

There are still some problems which have to be solved.

The voice obtained with our prosthesis is far superior to oesophageal speech since in most cases our patients can even sing! Several factors limit the potential of this voice, namely:

- pulmonary pressure
- tube resistance to air flow
- the oesophageal sphincter
- the pharynx.

We have not yet been able to determine precisely the role of each of these factors. The study of muscular contraction and its control should be carried out with electromyography during vocalization together with pressure and flow studies.

Correct voice production is guaranteed by controlling pressure, flow variations, and, in the case of laryngeal voice, muscles.

A better knowledge of all these relevant factors could contribute to practical advances in phoniatric rehabilitation and thus to improvements in the voice quality and personal comfort of laryngectomized patients.

The Anatomy of the Larynx, Pharynx and Cervical Oesophagus in Relation to Surgical Voice Restoration*

J. LANG [1]

1. Introduction

Any anatomical study of the remaining pharynx and oesophagus after laryngectomy must consider innervation and muscle fibre course. One hitherto unsolved problem is the simultaneous arrival of nerve impulses in the vocalis, pharynx and oesophagus muscles from the left and right. It is known that the left recurrent laryngeal nerve has to cover a longer distance than the right one. This is why the course of the nerve fibres from their nuclei to their effector organs needs to be briefly described. The motoric fibres of the vagus nerve emerge from the large-cell nucleus which is approximately 20 mm long and 3 mm thick. It stretches cranially from the region of the medullary stria and caudad until the decussation of the pyramids (Kirsch et al. 1968). The nucleus is approximately 4 mm below the floor of the fourth ventricle in cranial areas and about 6 mm deep in caudal areas. It is sited ventrally and somewhat laterally to the gracile nucleus. Fibres for the palatine and pharyngeal muscles go from a small rostral area into the glossopharyngeal and vagus nerves. Fibres for the larynx muscle go from the larger caudal section into nerve X. Fibres for the superior laryngeal nerve come from the rostral part of the laryngeal segment. Those for the cricoarytenoid muscles emerge from a somewhat more caudal area. Fibres for the arytenoid muscles emerge from an area placed even farther caudally (Kirsch 1968).

2. The Vagus Nerve

The axons of the large-cell nucleus form an inner knee within the central nervous organ. The course inside the brain stem until its emergence in the retro-olivaris area measures about 8.5 mm.

8.5 (4–15) rootlets from the vagus nerve enter the retro-olivaris area. Their glial segments are about 0.1 mm long where they run more medially and up to 2 mm where they run laterally (Lang 1982). Until their entry through the dural orifice, the uppermost and lowermost rootlets had a mean length of 15.33 mm and 15.60 mm, respectively (Lang and Reiter, to be published). Distal to the su-

* This work is dedicated to my colleague and dear friend Professor Dr. med. Walter Kley, head of the Department of Otolaryngology, University of Würzburg, on his 65th birthday.

[1] Anatomisches Institut der Universität Würzburg, Koellikerstraße 6, D-8700 Würzburg.

Speech Restoration Via Voice Prostheses
Edited by I. F. Herrmann

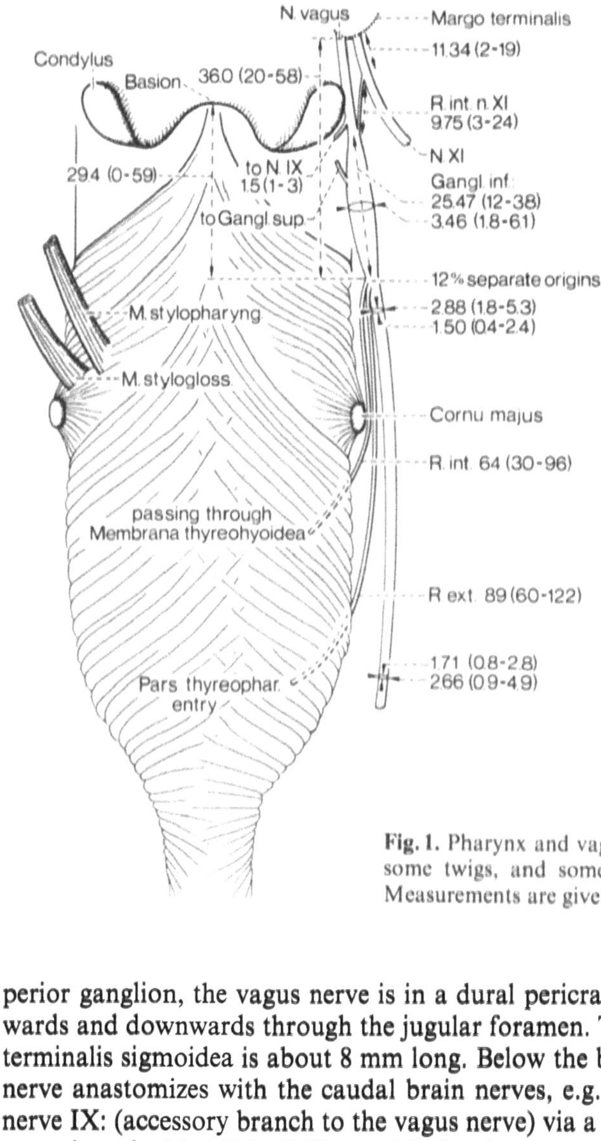

Fig. 1. Pharynx and vagus nerve (with inferior ganglion, some twigs, and some anastomoses) viewed dorsally. Measurements are given in mm (extremals)

perior ganglion, the vagus nerve is in a dural pericranium sheath and runs forwards and downwards through the jugular foramen. The stretch up to the crista terminalis sigmoidea is about 8 mm long. Below the base of the skull, the vagus nerve anastomizes with the caudal brain nerves, e.g., with the inner branch of nerve IX: (accessory branch to the vagus nerve) via a 9.75 (3–24) mm long anastomosis and with 1.5 (1–3) fibres with the glossopharyngeal nerve, together with the superior cervical ganglion and the ventral nerve ansa C1/C2 (Fig. 1). In our studies together with Vogel and Müller the inferior ganglion of nerve X was found to be 25.47 (12–38) mm long and 3.46 (1.8–6.1) mm thick. In our specimens, the distance between the crista terminalis and the lower edge of the inferior ganglion was 36.0 (20–58) mm. This is usually the zone in which the superior laryngeal nerve branches off. Despite great individual variations, the mean length of the total distance from the large-cell nucleus to the lower edge of the ganglion amounted to 68.1 mm. It is generally thought that the pericaria for the visceral afferent fibres (from the larynx, pharynx, viscera of the thorax and abdomen) are situated in the inferior ganglion of the vagus nerve. Similarly, it is thought that those fibres of the somatic system (auricular branch, recurrent laryngeal nerve, pharyngeal branches, meningeal branch) are found in the superior ganglion (Kerr 1962; Rhoton et al. 1966; Sobusiak et al. 1972/73 etc.).

3. The Superior Laryngeal Nerve (Fig. 2)

The superior laryngeal nerve usually branches off from the lower edge area of the inferior ganglion of the vagus nerve and runs for 21 (3–44) mm as a homogeneous stem. In 12% of our specimens, the internal branch and external branch had separate origins. Doubling of the external ramus was also noticed. In one specimen, Leichsenring and Hegener (1924) found a three-root external branch originating directly from the vagus nerve. The distance to the thyropharyngeal part of the pharyngeal constrictor was 89 (60–122) mm in our specimens. It was almost usual to find unions with the sympathetic trunk and the capsule of the thyroid gland

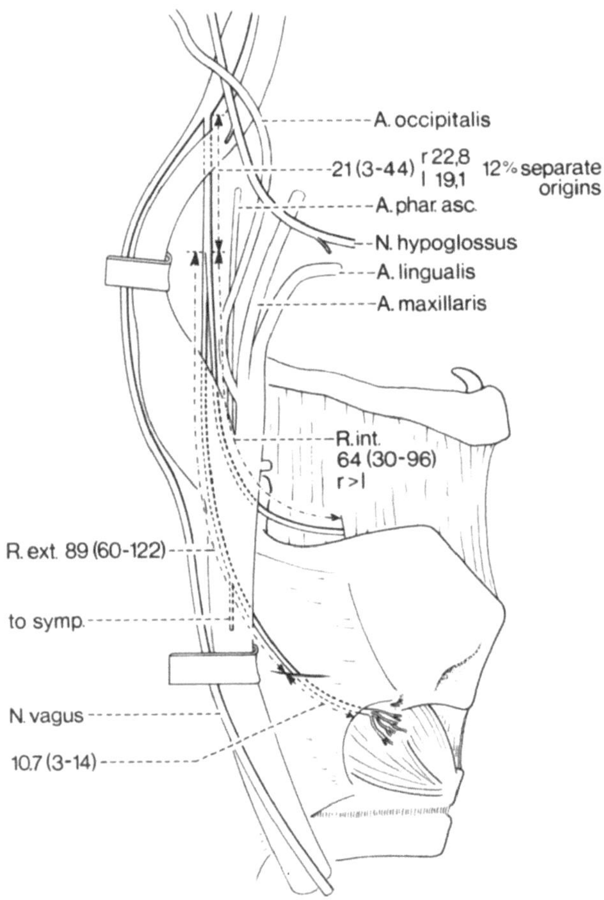

Fig. 2. Superior laryngeal nerve with external branch and internal branch, viewed laterally. Measurements in mm (extremals)

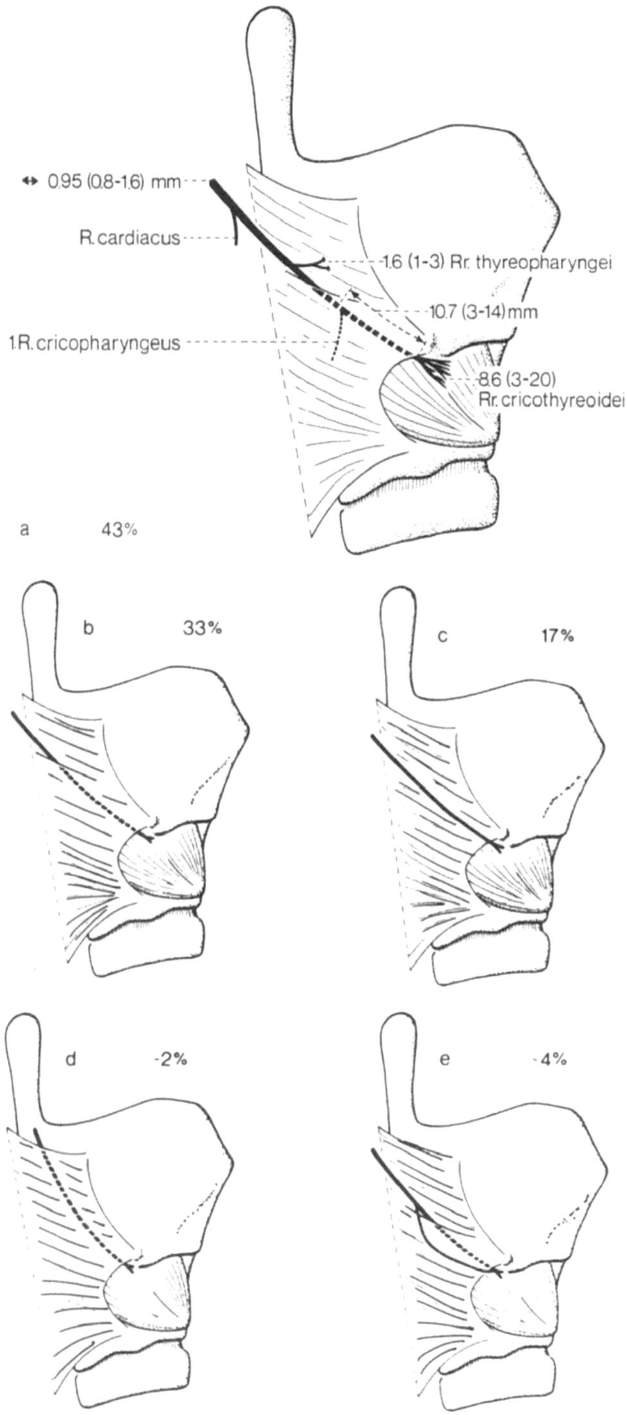

Fig. 3. a External branch, twigs and course in 43%. Measurements in mm (extremals). **b–e.** Course of the external branch of the superior laryngeal nerve to the thyreopharyngeal part of the inferior pharyngeal constrictor

or with the cardiac branches of the external branch. Therefore, the overall mean length of the nerve between the large-cell nerve and the thyropharyngeal part was 178.1 mm (mean value) for our specimens.

External Branch; Branches to the Inferior Constrictor Muscle of the Pharynx. In our specimens, 1.6 (1–3) thyropharyngeal branches went off to the muscle part of the same name and one cricopharyngeal branch went off to the lowest part of the inferior constrictor muscle of the pharynx.

In 43% of cases, the external branch (Fig. 3) penetrates the thyropharyngeal part and runs below it for about 10.7 (3–14) mm before dividing into 8.6 (3–20) branches leading to the cricothyroid muscle. Some of these nerve fibres pass through the muscle and reach the inside of the larynx. In 33% of cases, the nerve runs below for nearly the whole of the thyropharyngeal part. In 17% of cases, the nerve runs along the surface. In about 2% of cases, it completely twigs in below this muscle section. Finally, in about 4% of cases, one branch was found below and one branch on the surface of the muscle.

4. The Recurrent Laryngeal Nerve (Fig. 4)

Directly below the inferior ganglion of the vagus nerve, this nerve including its perineurium and connective tissue, was found to be 2.88 (1.8–5.3) mm wide and

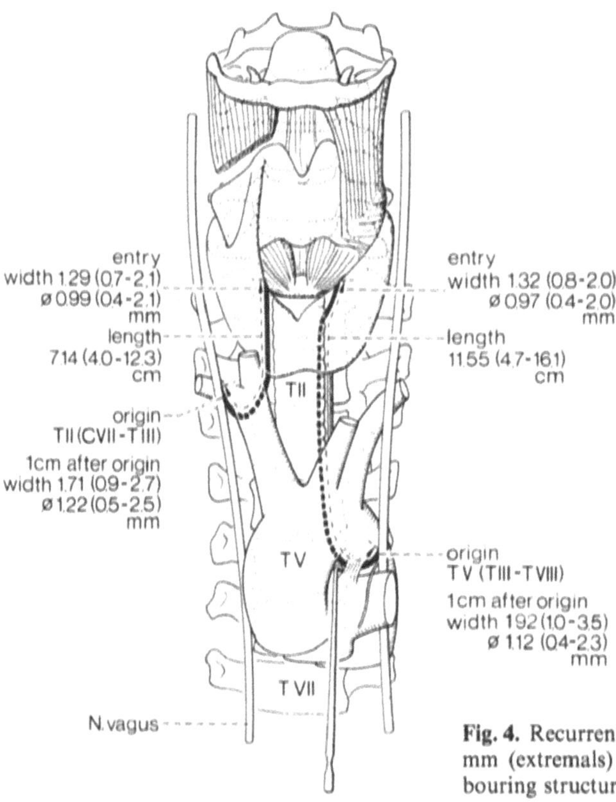

Fig. 4. Recurrent laryngeal nerves in cm and mm (extremals) and their relation to neighbouring structures

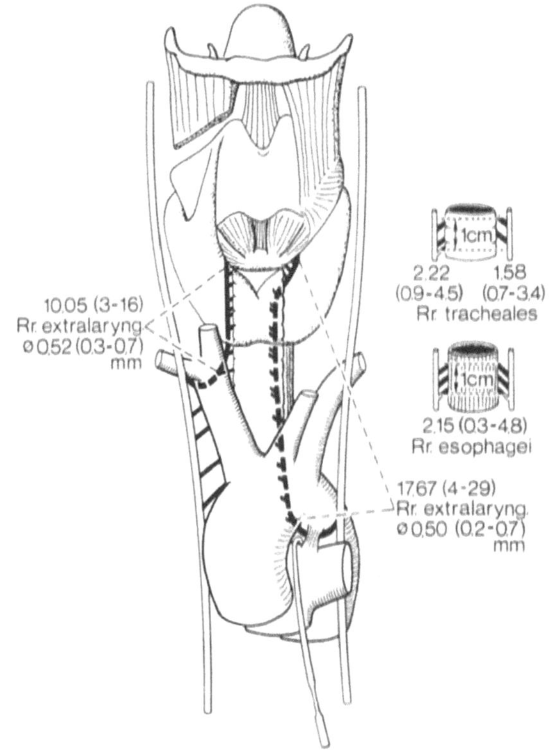

Fig. 5. Recurrent laryngeal nerves, extralaryngeal twigs to trachea and oesophagus. Diameters in mm (extremals) and numbers of twigs

1.50 (0.4–2.4) mm thick. Farther in a distal direction, it was 2.66 (0.9–4.9) mm wide and 1.71 (0.8–2.8) mm thick. On average, the right recurrent laryngeal nerve usually divides in the lower area of the second thoracic vertebra (from C7 to mid – T3). The left one usually divides in the upper third of the fifth thoracic vertebra (T3 to T8). The mean length of the left and right sides of the recurrent laryngeal nerve until its entry into the pharynx was 7.14 (4.0–12.3) cm and 11.55 (4.7–16.1) cm, respectively.

Figure 4 shows the thickness (including perineural sheaths) of the recurrent nerves. It also shows the way the course of the right recurrent laryngeal nerve tends more to the oesophagotracheal angle. Outside the larynx in our specimens, 10.05 (3–16) branches were found on the right to the oesophagus and trachea and 17.67 (4–29) on the left with diameters of 0.50 (0.2–0.7) mm. Figure 5 shows the branches going to the trachea and oesophagus (1 centimeter long areas). Before the recurrent laryngeal nerve reaches its point of entry, we found in about 70% of our specimens that the nerve runs dorsally to the lateral suspensory ligament of the thyroid gland and more frequently on the right than on the left. In 4.7% of cases, it runs ventrally to this thyroid gland ligament. In 26% of cases, it runs through the ligament (more frequently on the right than the left).

The Recurrent Laryngeal Nerve; Entry into the Larynx (Fig. 6). In our specimens, 1.8 (1–4) and 1.62 (1–4) branches went to the right and the left of the pharyngo-oesophageal junction. Most frequently, 2 branches were found where the one run-

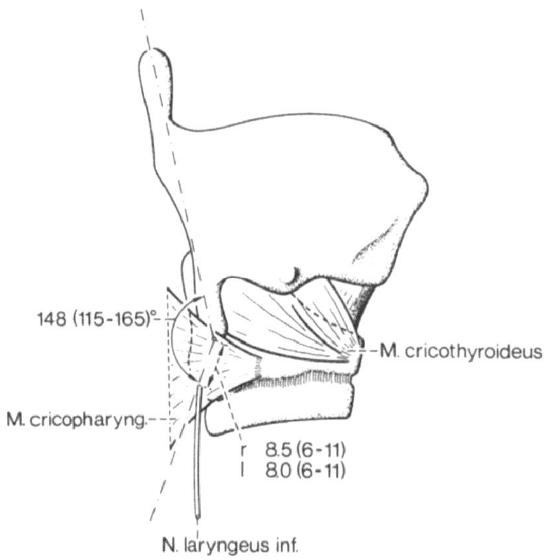

Fig. 6. Entrance zone of the inferior laryngeal nerve into the inferior horn of the thyroid cartilage. Measurements in mm and degrees (extremals)

ning more dorsally connected with the internal branch of the superior laryngeal nerve. In 63% of cases, the muscular branch of the nerve penetrates the cricopharyngeal part. The others penetrate the oesophago-tracheal corner laterally and below the cricopharyngeal part. The entry zone is 8.5 (6–11) mm to the right and 8.0 (6–11) mm to the left of the inferior horn of the thyroid cartilage. The angle between the inferior horn of the thyroid cartilage and the entry zone of the nerve was 148 ° (115–165 °). This means that the nerve can be found farther dorsally (115 °) or even almost below the inferior horn of the thyroid cartilage (165 °).

5. The Course of the Nerve in the Larynx (Fig. 7)

After entering the larynx, the recurrent laryngeal nerve is known as the inferior laryngeal nerve. It divides into a posterior branch, which runs to the posterior cricoarytenoid and arytenoid muscles, and into an anterior branch, which supplies the lateral cricoarytenoid, thyroarytenoid, and vocalis muscles. After its entry into the larynx and prior to its branching, the inferior laryngeal nerve is 1.38 (0.69–2.08) mm wide and 0.99 (0.39–2.08) mm thick. It must be emphasized that these measurements were carried out by Lang, Fischer and Nachbaur on specimens under the stereoscopic microscope and that only diameters of 332.86 (53.4–534.0) µm were derived in histological specimens for pure nerve cross sections.

Except for the branch of the ansa galeni, the posterior branch normally divides off behind and above the cricothyroid joint. This branch runs beneath the posterior cricothyroid muscle supplying it with 6.22 (1–12) branches whose average width and thickness are 0.22 mm and 0.16 mm, respectively. 1.74 (1–5) and 5.29 (1–10) of these branches are absorbed by the lateral region and ventral surface of this muscle, respectively. The end branch of the posterior ramus is the branch of the arytenoid muscle (Ramus m. artenoidei) which runs upwards for

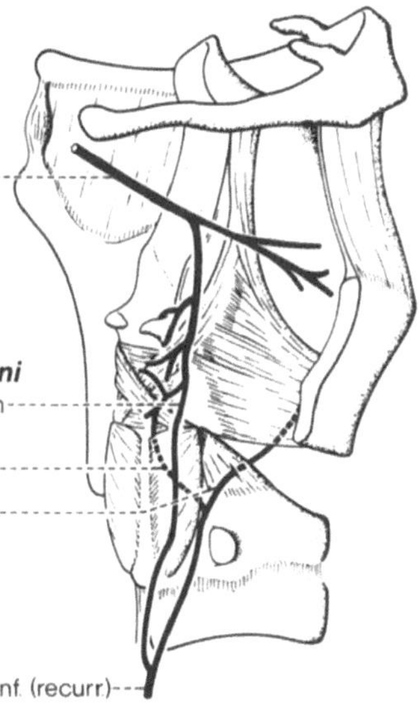

Fig. 7. The most common intralaryngeal course of the inferior and superior laryngeal nerves and ansa galeni

10.8 (8–14) mm below the posterior crico-arytenoid muscle and supplies the transverse arytenoid muscle with 1.5 (1–3) branches. The transverse diameter and thickness of these arytenoid branches were 0.42 (0.17–1.05 mm) and 0.22 (0.06–0.48) mm, respectively.

The anterior branch divides into an average of 3.54 (2–6) lateral cricoarytenoid branches whose transverse diameter and thickness were 0.27 (0.13–0.57) mm and 0.21 (0.12–0.42) mm, respectively. We observed 2.06 (1–5) branches leading to the thyroarytenoid muscles whose diameter and thickness were 0.38 (0.09–1.20) mm and 0.23 (0.09–0.48) mm, respectively.

The Ansa Galeni (Figs. 7, 8, and 9)

The ansa galeni is 7.36 (5.6–9.6) cm long between its exit from the recurrent laryngeal nerve and the superior laryngeal nerve. We found its width (including sheath tissue) and thickness were 0.87 (0.36–1.8) mm and 0.43 (0.21–0.90) mm, respectively. At its exit from the recurrent laryngeal nerve, its transverse diameter and thickness were only 0.48 (0.21–0.90) mm and 0.34 (0.18–0.60) mm, respectively. Microscopical studies of specimens have determined that 4.5 (3–13) branches divide off from the ansa which then divide further. After splitting, 13.3 (1–24) branches find their way to mucous membrane and 3.67 (1–8) to various muscles. Moreover, there were additional anastomoses with branches of the superior and inferior laryngeal nerves in 50% of cases. The ansa galeni itself was found in 54.4% of cases. See Fig. 8 for further possible anastomoses. In about one third of the cases, no unions could be found between the laryngeal nerves. It should be emphasized that, like Dilworth (1921/22), Morrison (1952), Keros and Nemanić (1967), we usually found the ramifications of the branch for the ansa galeni from the recurrent laryngeal nerve 2.5 cm below the cricoid cartilage.

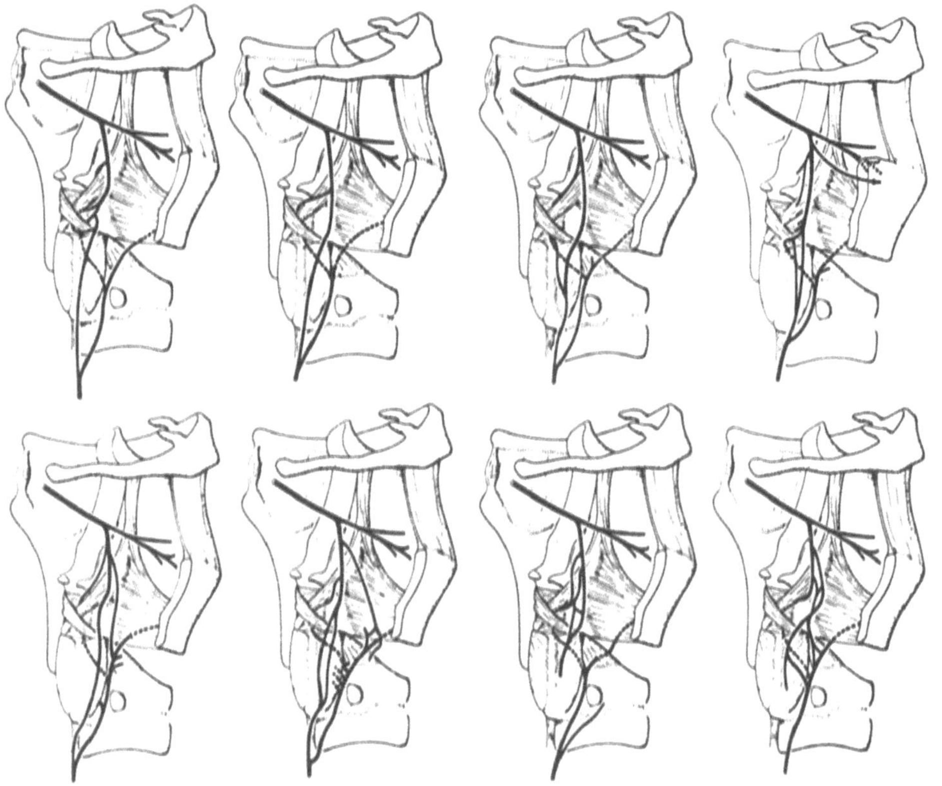

Fig. 8. Variations of the ansa galeni and the twigs of the internal laryngeal nerves

6. The Problem of Nerve Impulses Arriving at the Larynx and Pharynx Muscles

In our cases, the right and left recurrent laryngeal nerves were 7.14 and 11.55 cm long between the exit from the vagus nerve and entrance into the larynx. The difference would therefore seem to be only 4.41 cm. However, it must be emphasized that in our studies (mainly old people) the fibres of the left recurrent laryngeal nerve ran on average almost 3 vertebrae (and discs) farther caudad than the right one. Only this would explain the findings of Krmpotić (1958) that there was a lateral difference of 10 (5.7–15) cm in length between the left and right recurrent laryngeal nerve. Shin and Rabuzzi (1971) also found a difference in length of 11 cm. According to Krmpotić (1958), the nerve fibres between the nuclear area and the arytenoid muscle are 32.2 cm on the right and 42.6 cm on the left. At the entrance into the larynx (see Fig. 4), we found that the left recurrent laryngeal nerve was 1.32 mm wide. The right one was 1.29 mm and also had a larger transverse diameter. This does not mean that more numerous or thicker fibres are to be found in the left recurrent laryngeal nerve. Under the microscope, Krmpotić also found fibre thicknesses of 7.3 (2–11) μm on the left and 5.4 (1–9) μm on the right which

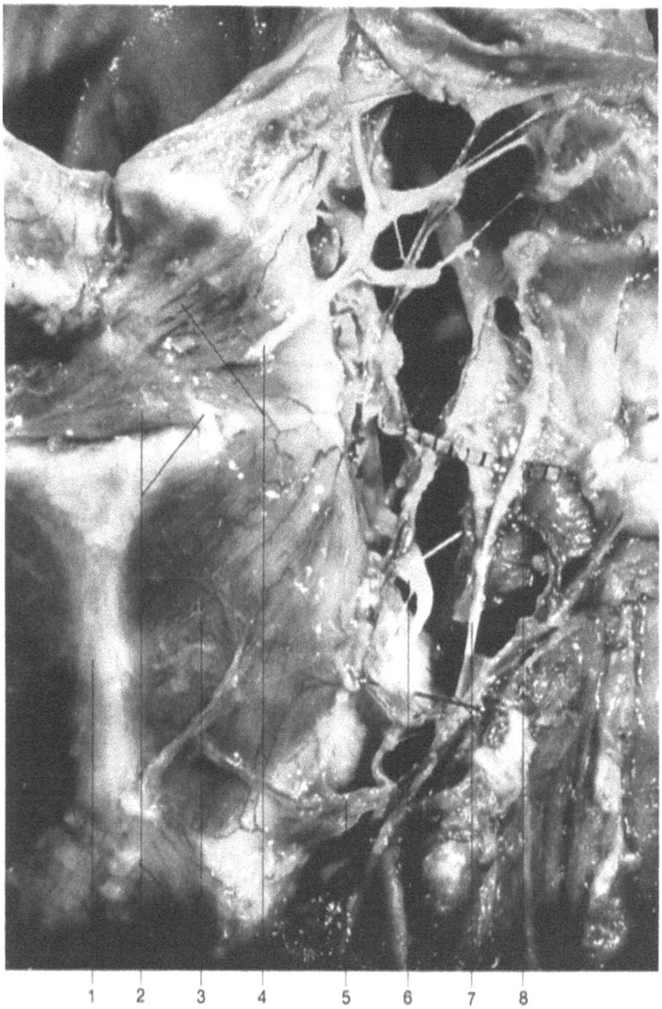

Fig. 9. Nerves and vessels on the posterior surface of the larynx: *1*, Cricoid cartilage, medial crest. *2*, Arytenoid muscle and twig of the inferior laryngeal nerve. *3*, Posterior cricoarytenoid muscle. *4*, Oblique arytenoid muscle and twig of the superior laryngeal nerve. *5*, Twig of the inferior laryngeal artery. *6*, Dorsal branch of the inferior laryngeal nerve. *7*, Facies artic. inf. of the cricoid cartilage and twig of the inferior laryngeal nerve to the mucous membrane. *8*, Cricopharyngeal part (ascending) of the constrictor pharyngis fixed laterally (mm paper)

could point to the left recurrent laryngeal nerve having a quicker pathway. According to Abdallah and King (1979), however, 43% more myelinated fibres occur in the right recurrent laryngeal nerve than in the left, while Gacek and Lyon (1976) state that the former also has more fibres. Malmgren and Gacek (1981) found in this nerve that only 12.4 (6.0–30.0) % of 1 to 11 nerve fasciculi were included in a cross section of the nerve. They histochemically subdivided nerve fibres into a Group I where diameters were about 7.9 μm and took up a surface area of 0.17 ± 0.004 mm^2 in the nerve cross section. They also reacted with acetylcholinesterase. Apart from these, there were also thinner fibres of 3.2 and 3.6 μm which reacted in the same way. It was assumed that Group I fibres would take over muscle supply whilst Group II fibres with thicknesses of 7.6 μm showed no reaction and were possibly sensory. In all, it seems that the problem of nerve impulses arriving simultaneously at the larynx and pharynx has still not been solved. It is well known that Holzapfel (1899) found 3 non-recurrent recurrent laryngeal nerves. They wound around anomalous arterial origins. Another 4 ran round the right vertebral artery which was a branch of the right common carotid artery. Williams (1933) compiled 28 such cases. Pemberton and Miller (1941) also found non-recurrent recurrent laryngeal nerves during operations. It is much rarer to find non-recurrent left laryngeal nerves, namely, when the 4th, 5th and 6th arch artery is stunted and the nerve has not been displaced caudad.

7. Pharyngo-Oesophageal Junction; Muscles

Knowledge of the pharyngo-oesophageal junction area and its variants, which have been neglected in most textbooks, is of medical interest for the insertion of voice prostheses.

a) Thyropharyngeal Part

The thyropharyngeal part usually starts not only at the oblique line but also in an area of varying width at the thyroid cartilage. In our specimens, we frequently found junctions from the sternothyroid muscle into the thyropharyngeal part. In 43% of specimens, we found origins of inferior thyroid cartilage tubercle.

b) Cricopharyngeal Part (Fig. 10)

Waldeyer (1927) differentiated five different types of origin for the cricopharyngeal part. Among other things, he also noticed muscular connections between the cricothyroid muscle and the cricopharyngeal part, intermediary tendons between both muscles, tendinous arches, spanning the cricothyroid muscle and serving the middle part of the inferior constrictor muscle of the pharynx as a zone of origin, as well as the inferior constrictor muscle of the pharynx overlapping the cricothy-

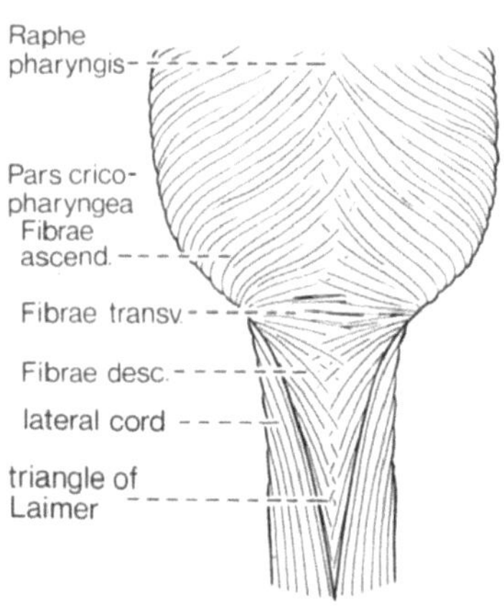

Fig. 10. Oesophagopharyngeal junction, viewed dorsally

roid muscle. In about 54% of our specimens, the cricothyroid muscle gives off fibres to the inferior constrictor muscle of the pharynx. In the remaining specimens, both muscles could be isolated from each other. We calculate that the potential force development of the cricopharyngeal part is 12.30 (6.0–26.0) N. In the cricopharyngeal part, we differentiated ascending fibres running backwards and upwards, transverse fibres and descending fibres. The transverse fibres represent the sphincter mechanism of the oesophageal orifice. Batson (1956) observed thickenings of this transverse muscle fibre layer of up to 12 mm, which we also sometimes found in our specimens. One assumes that a special state of contraction, caused by defective innervation of this nerve part, may produce dysphagia. Blakeley et al. (1968) therefore proposed that the cricopharyngeal part can be transsected. Pressures at this sphincter level are 20–30 cm H_2O higher than in the upper oesophagus. Weihrauch et al. (1980) found in 119 healthy patients (20–49 years) pressures of 144.4 ± 8.6 mm Hg. In patients between fifty and eighty years old they found pressures of 103.4 ± 4.2 Hg. It is a known fact that dysphagies can also be caused by neoplasms, paralysis of the pharyngeal constrictor muscle, muscular dystrophies, thyrotoxicoses, myasthenia gravis, osteophytes of the anterior aspect of the cervical vertebral column. During deglutition, the cricopharyngeal part relaxes for less than one second immediately before the superior constrictor muscle of the pharynx contracts. These processes are governed by a reflex arc centred in the floor area of the fourth ventricle (Chodosch 1975). The afferences run in the glossopharyngeal and vagus nerves from proprioceptors as well as from sympathetic and parasympathetic fibres in the pharyngeal plexus. The efferences mainly come from the large-cell nucleus. According to Hampton (1960), the sympathetic nerve governs the relaxation and the vagus nerve controls the contraction of the inferior constrictor muscle of the pharynx. In one of his cases, a pharyngeal diverticulum developed after a cricopharyngeal dysphagia.

According to Zenker and Zenker (1960), the ascending fibres of the cricopharyngeal (and thyropharyngeal) parts make the upper part of the cricoid cartilage lamina tip forward thereby producing a contraction of the vocal chord. Minnigerode (1967) thinks this is unlikely. The descending fibres of the cricopharyngeal part (variably formed) radiate backwards, downwards, and medially into Laimer's trigone (see Fig. 10).

c) Origin of Oesophagus

The cranial origin of oesophageal longitudinal muscle occurs at the dorsal median of the cricoid lamina via a ligamentous apparatus of varying length: the crico-oesophageal ligament. The muscle fibre bundles diverge in a downward direction. They grasp the back of Laimer's trigone from a lateral position downwards (Fig. 9). After freeing the laryngeal skeleton and the trachea, we showed these lateral muscle bounds from the front. Muscle fibres from the lower edge of the cricoid cartilage run for varying lengths in a cranial direction (0.0–13) mm (Fig. 11). In one case, the right origin was 3 mm higher than the left one. In another case, the left origin was 5 mm higher than the right one. The circular eal muscle fibres layer of the oesophagus begins at the lower edge area of the cricoid cartilage carmina. If one frees the cricopharyngeal part and moves it laterally the

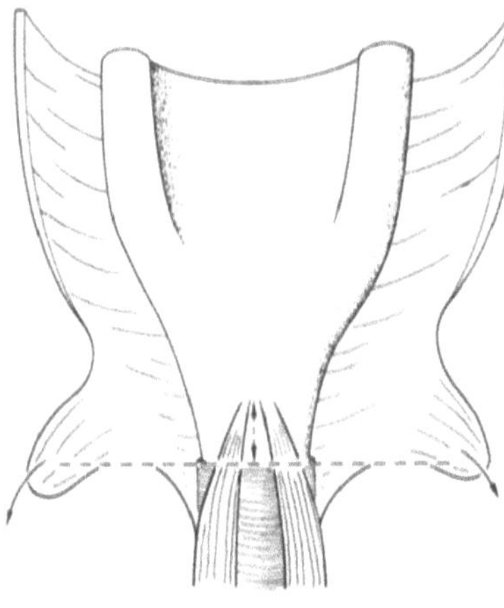

11 r 6,5 (0-13) l 6,7 (0-13)

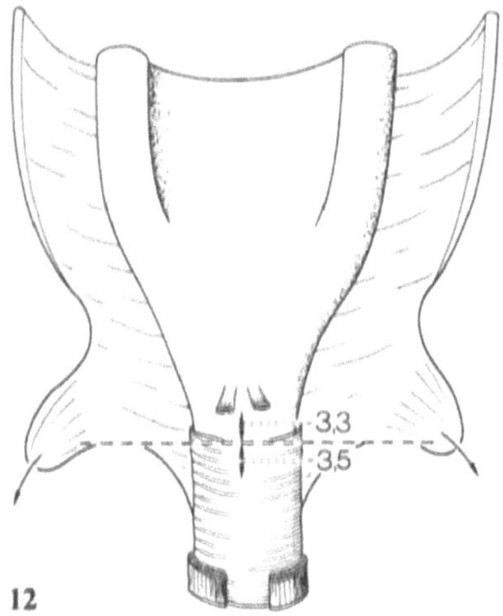

12

Fig. 11. Origin of the most important longitudinal oesophageal fibres in relation to the lower border of the cricopharyngeal muscle. Viewed from the front after resection of the larynx, measurements in mm (extremals)

Fig. 12. Site of the uppermost circular muscle fibres of the oesophagus in relation to the lower border of the cricopharyngeal part of the inferior pharyngeal constrictor. Viewed from the front after resection of the larynx

cricoid fibre area reaches up to 3.3 mm and up to 3.5 mm above and below the lower edge of the cricopharyngeal part, respectively. In half of our specimens, the lateral muscle belly had to be removed so that the cricoid fibre layer could be seen. In the remaining specimens, it was visible in the central area without any further removals (Fig. 12).

Like us, Laimer (1883) found in about 5% of cases a 2–3 cm long muscle bundle branching off from the lower edge of the cricoid cartilage below the cricothyroid joint and settling on the lateral muscle bundle. The recurrent laryngeal nerve and the inferior laryngeal artery enter the pharyngo-oesophageal junction dorsal to the muscle bundle. It must be emphasized that fibres can also go from the area of the palatopharyngeus muscle into the longitudinal oesophageal muscle. This was first pointed out by Cleland and Mackay (1896) and then later by Abel (1913).

Even the old anatomists, e.g., Luschka (1862) knew that the oesophagus usually seems somewhat dilated and more so to the left than to the right. In our specimens, it stretched for 2.49 (0–7.1) cm. The oesophagus protrudes 3.98 (1.2–10.3) cm past the lateral margins of the trachea and more to the left than the right. The oesophagus extended 0.81 (0.4–1.6) cm and 0.47 (0.02–0.8) cm past the side of the trachea on the left and right, respectively. The lateral difference is statistically significant (t-value).

8. Nerve Stimulation

Even Berendes (1956) emphasized that the question had been discussed for a long time as to whether, besides the cricothyroid muscle and other exterior muscles, the superior laryngeal nerve plays a part in the innervation of the inner laryngeal muscles and especially the arytenoid muscle. Fabbi (1948) was the first one to stimulate the nerve and never noticed any contractions of the arytenoid muscle. However, this muscle contracted regularly when stimulated by the recurrent laryngeal nerve. Williams (1951) agreed with this (quotation of Mündnich 1956). Mündnich (1956) emphasizes that a sphincter-like reflex occurs when the superior laryngeal nerve is stimulated. On the other hand, the arytenoid muscle and the posterior cricoarytenoid muscle were not seen to contract after the reflexes had been stopped and the recurrent laryngeal nerves transsected. Electrophysiological investigations of the recurrent laryngeal nerve were obviously first carried out on human beings by Mündnich. Strong stimulation produced a sphincter-like closure of the glottis. By contrast, Rethi (1969) is of the opinion that small laryngeal muscles possess twin innervation. He believes that the main innervator is the recurrent laryngeal nerve, the superior laryngeal nerve being responsible for the tonic contraction of the abductors and the adductors. Peytz et al. (1965) as well as Atkins (1973) point out that the rate of conduction is the same in both of the recurrent laryngeal nerves (on average 65 m/s). They claim that it is slower in distal nerve sections than in proximal ones. Shin and Rabuzzi (1971) supramaximally stimulated dog recurrent nerves and made recordings via muscle electrodes in the larynx. They found the rate of conduction for the right recurrent laryngeal nerve was 2.7 ± 0.5 m/s. Over a middle distance it was 9.6 ± 1.0 cm. The left recurrent laryngeal nerve had a rate of conduction of 2.8 ± 0.3 m/s over a distance of 9.0 ± 1.0 cm. This would mean that the right and left recurrent laryngeal nerves have an average rate of conduction of 35.7 m/s and 32.2 m/s, respectively. However, their findings do indicate that there is a higher rate of conduction in the proximal part of the left recurrent nerve than in the right one. The authors attribute this to the higher thickness of the fibres of the left nerve (as Krmpotić 1956, has presumed).

Conclusions

1. During laryngectomy with preservation of the pharynx muscles, one must consider the numerous variations of the inferior constrictor muscle of the pharynx including the possibility of a thickened transverse part of the cricopharyngeal part. It seems important to know the lateral muscle cords as origins of longitudinal oesophagus muscle. It also seems important to know their origin on the cricoid lamina.

2. The inferior constrictor muscle of the pharynx is mainly innervated from the external branch of the superior laryngeal nerve. It branches off at varying heights from the superior laryngeal nerve and (in 12% of cases) from the inferior ganglion itself. The anatomical course and the entry region of the recurrent laryngeal nerve as well as its branches to the oesophagus and pharyngo-oesophageal junction should be preserved untouched. This will keep the innervation of the remaining part of the pharynx.

References

Abdalla AB, King AS (1979) Afferent and efferent myelinated fibres in branches of the avian vagus. J Anat 129:69–75
Abel W (1913) The arrangement of the longitudinal and circular musculature at the upper end of the oesophagus. J Anat Physiol 47:381–390
Batson OV (1956) The cricopharyngeus muscle. Ann Otol 64:47–54
Berendes J (1956) Neuere Ergebnisse über Bewegungsstörungen des Kehlkopfes. Arch Ohren-, Nasen- und Kehlkopfheilkunde 169:1–172
Blakeley WR et al. (1968) Section of the cricopharyngeus muscle for dysphagia. Arch Surg 96:745–762
Chodosh PL (1975) Cricopharyngeal myotomy in the treatment of dysphagia. Laryngoscope 85:1862–1873
Cleland M (1913) cited from Abel (1913)
Dilworth TF (1921/22) The nerves of the human larynx. J Anat 56:48–52
Fabbi (1948) cited from Berendes (1956)
Gacek RR, Lyon MJ (1976) Fiber components of the recurrent laryngeal nerve in the cat. Ann Otol 85:460–471
Hamptom J (1960) Cricopharyngeal dysphagia. Am J Roentgenol, Rad Therapy and Nucl Med 84:1028–1036
Holzapfel G (1899) Ungewöhnlicher Ursprung und Verlauf der Arteria subclavia dextra. Anat Hefte 12:373–376
Keros P, Nemanić D (1967) The terminal branching of the recurrent laryngeal nerve. Pract Oto-Rhino-Laryng 29:5–10
Kerr FW (1962) Facial, vagal and glossopharyngeal nerves in the cat. Arch Neurol 6:264–281
Kirsch WM et al. (1968) Laryngeal palsy in association with myelomeningocele, hydrocephalus and the Arnold-Chiari malformation. J Neurosurg 28:297–314
Krmpotić J (1956) Über den wahren Verlauf des rechten Nervus recurrens. Arch Ohren-, Nasen- und Kehlkopfheilkunde 169:533–539
Krmpotić J (1958) Anatomisch-histologische und funktionelle Verhältnisse des rechten und des linken Nervus recurrens mit Rücksicht auf die Geschwindigkeit der Impulsleitung bei einer Ursprungsanomalie der rechten Schlüsselbeinarterie. Arch Ohren-, Nasen- und Kehlkopfheilkunde 173:490–496
Laimer E (1883) Beitrag zur Anatomie des Oesophagus. Wiener Med Jahrbuch 333–385
Lang J (1982) Über Bau, Länge und Gefäßbeziehungen der „zentralen" und „peripheren" Strekken der intrazisternalen Hirnnerven. Ein Beitrag zur vaskulären Hirnnervenschädigung und Dekompressionsbehandlung bei Trigeminusneuralgie, okulärer Neuromyotomie, Spasmus hemifacialis, Tinnitus und Vertigo, Glossopharyngeusneuralgie und Caput obstipum spasticum. Zbl Neurochirurgie 43:217–258
Lang J, Reiter U (to be published) Über die intrazisternale Länge der Nn. VII–XII. Neurochirurgia
Lang J, Fischer K, Nachbaur St, Meuer H-W (1986) Über den Verlauf und die Zweige des N. laryngeus recurrens, der A. thyreoidea inferior und der A. laryngea inferior. Gegenbaurs Morph Jahrb 132:617–643
Lang J, Nachbaur St, Fischer K (1986) Nn. laryngei, Verzweigungen im Kehlkopfinneren. Gegenbaurs Morph Jahrb 132:723–736
Lang J, Nachbaur St, Fischer K (to be published) N. laryngei, Verzweigungen im Kehlkopfinneren. Gegenbaurs Morph Jahrb
Leichsenring E, Hegener J (1924) Die curative Recurrenslähmung und das Rosenbach-Semonsche Gesetz. Z Hals-Nasen-Ohrenheilkunde 7:284–313
Luschka H von (1862) Die Anatomie des menschlichen Halses. 1. Band, 1. Abteilung. Lauppsche Buchhandlung, Tübingen
Malmgren LT, Gacek RR (1981) Acetylcholinesterase staining of fiber components in feline and human recurrent laryngeal nerve. Acta Otolaryngol 91:337–352
Minnigerode B (1967) Untersuchungen zur Bedeutung der extralaryngealen Muskulatur für den Phonationsakt unter besonderer Berücksichtigung des Musculus cricopharyngeus. Arch Klin Exp Ohren-, Nasen- und Kehlkopfheilkunde 188:604–623

Morrison LF (1952) Recurrent laryngeal nerve paralysis. A revised conception based on the dissection of one hundred cadavers. Ann Otol 61:567–592
Mündnich K (1956) Anatomische und histologische Untersuchungen und Experimente zur Physiologie und Pathologie des menschlichen Kehlkopfes. Arch Ohren-, Nasen- und Kehlkopfheilkunde 169:190–196
Pemberton J de, Miller JM (1941) Anomaly of the right inferior laryngeal nerve. Arch Surg 42:712–718
Peytz F et al. (1965) Conduction time and velocity in human recurrent laryngeal nerve. Danish Med Bull 12:125
Réthi A (1969) Innervations-Muskeltätigkeit, Stimmbildung. Arch Klin Exp Ohren-, Nasen- und Kehlkopfheilkunde 194:263–264
Rhoton AL et al. (1966) The trigeminal, facial and glossopharyngeal nerves in the monkey. Arch Neurol 14:530–539
Shin T, Rabuzzi DD (1971) Conduction studies of the canine recurrent laryngeal nerve. Laryngoscope 81:586–596
Sobusiak T et al. (1972/73) Primary glossopharyngeal and vagal efferent projection into the cerebellum in the dog. An experimental study with toluidine blue and silver impregnation methods. J Hirnforsch 13:117–136
Waldeyer A (1927) Zur Individual- und Rassenanatomie des menschlichen Kehlkopfes. Z Morph Anthropol 26:68–126
Weihrauch TR et al. (1980) Assessment of various factors influencing esophageal pressure measurement. Klin Wschr 58:279–292
Williams DG (1933) Anomaly of the inferior laryngeal nerve. Ann Surg 97:828–830
Williams AF (1951) The nerve supply of the laryngeal muscles. J Laryngol 15:343
Zenker W, Zenker A (1960) Über die Regelung der Stimmlippenspannung durch von außen eingreifende Mechanismen. Folia Phoniat 12:1–36

Glottoplasty with Functional Pharynx Surgery and Tracheostomaplasty

I. F. HERRMANN [1]

Introduction

The use of this improved primary technique will avoid the problems encountered with hypopharynx puncture. The problem is: Obtaining the right indication for performing the primary technique. Preoperative and postoperative lung function tests and preoperative check-ups have revealed that the primary technique can always be carried out when the results of the above tests and checks allow a laryngectomy to be made. The technique does not impede the learning of oesophageal speech. Contrary to the functional pharynx surgery facilitates the learning of oesophageal speech. In variance to the findings of Manni et al. (this volume, p. 33), we do not consider subglottic tumor extension and postcricoidal tumor growth to be contraindications of a primary voice restoration.

The Instrumental Set

The skin adhesive silicon stencil is used to mark the skin excision in order to facilitate a uniformly shaped tracheostoma. The universal puncture needle with handle is used to create the shunt between the respiratory tract and the upper digestive tract (Fig. 1). The inserter and its bullet-moulded end are coated with gel before insertion into the stent. The silicon stent of the voice prosthesis with its external and conic retention collar is introduced into the shunt during glottoplasty, hypopharynx-puncture and during radiation therapy. The voice prosthesis comes in two different sizes. The prosthesis is curved in order to shorten the distance between the valve and the open pharynx. It must be situated axially parallel in the digestive tract. These prostheses reduce the length of the collapsed pharynx and therefore also the pressure needed to open it. The prosthesis is held by a conic retention collar which, together with the tracheal plate cone, retains the prosthesis in the digestive tract. A guiding stick is used to insert the prosthesis into the shunt.

[1] Universitätsklinik und Poliklinik für Hals-, Nasen- und Ohrenkranke im Kopfklinikum, D-8700 Würzburg.

Speech Restoration Via Voice Prostheses
Edited by I. F. Herrmann

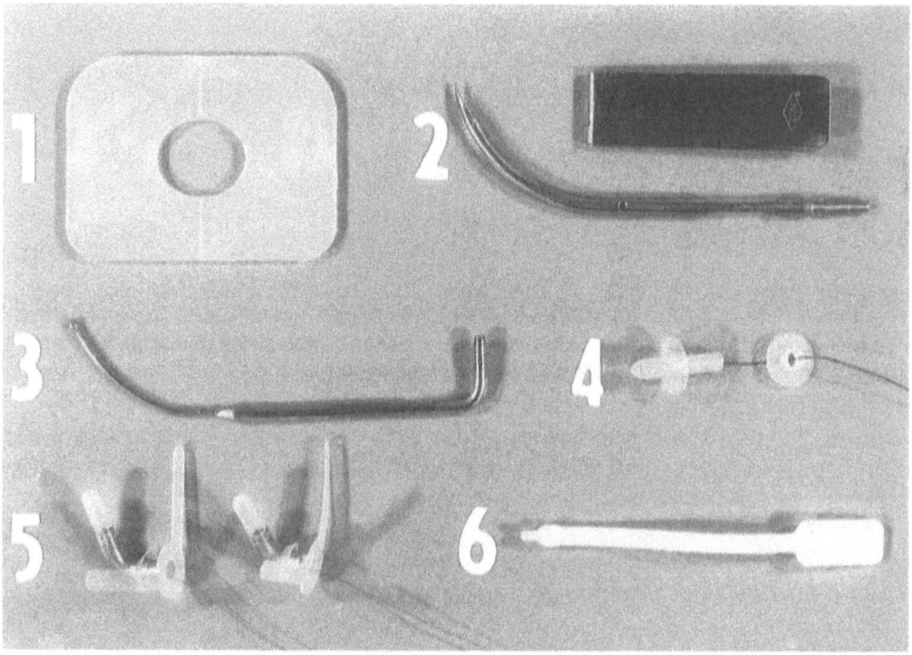

Fig. 1. The instrumental set: *1*, skin adhesive silicon stencil; *2*, universal puncture needle with handle; *3*, the inserter; *4*, the silicon stent of the voice prosthesis; *5*, the voice prostheses; *6*, the guiding stick for inserting the prosthesis

The Surgical Procedure

The surgical procedures are enumerated in steps 1 to 17. For the purposes of clarity, the surgical steps are divided into three stages: functional pharynx surgery, tracheostomaplasty and shunt surgery.

Skin incision; preparation of the platysma-fascia flap; division of the thyroid isthmus (after neck dissection and preparation of the larynx); lateral displacement of the thyroid flaps as well as tumor resection are known surgical procedures which do not need to be discussed here. In the paries membranaceus of the trachea a caudally pediculated mucosal flap (1.5 cm long) is peritomized prior to tumor removal (Step 3).

a) Glottoplasty with Functional Pharynx Surgery

We propose the following procedure to maintain muscle function, achieve better modulation and to produce effortless voice production: The cranial laryngeal nerve should be identified on both sides by using electrostimulation. In cases of radical tumor surgery the external nerve branches are only to be preserved (Step 1) if possible (Fig. 2). The thyreopharyngeal and cricopharyngeal muscles are cut at their origin in the thyroid and cricoid cartilage (Step 2).

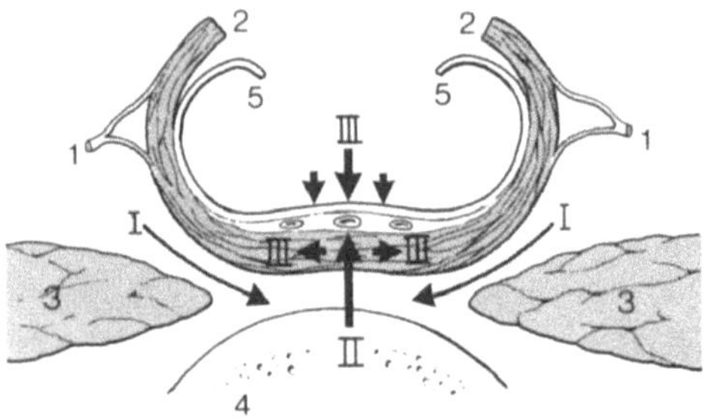

Fig. 2. Functional pharynx surgery. *I*, After laryngeal resection; the prevertebral region of the pharynx is mobilized bluntly. *II*, The constrictor musculature is separated dorso-medially. *III*, The dorsal muscle stumps are pushed bluntly to the side. *1*, The external branch of the cranial laryngeal nerve; *2*, the muscle stumps of the lower constrictor musculature; *3*, the prevertebral musculature; *4*, the vertebra; *5*, the pharyngeal mucosa

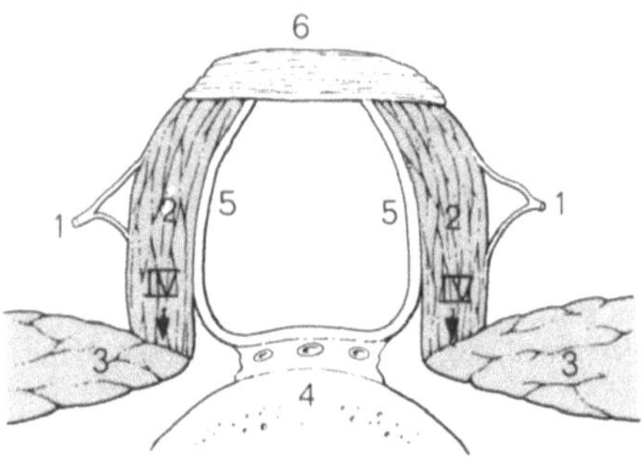

Fig. 3. Functional pharynx surgery. *IV*, After sealing the pharyngeal mucosa and the prevertebral tissue with fibrin tissue glue, the dorsal muscle stumps are sutured paramedially onto the prevertebral musculature 1 cm. The platysma fascia flap (*6*) is sewn above the laryngeal mucosa (*5*) and the laryngeal muscles attachments (*2*)

After laryngeal resection, the prevertebral region of the pharynx is mobilized bluntly (Step 5). The pharynx is turned to one side and the lower constrictor musculature is separated dorso-medially down to shunt level (Step 6a). We use magnifying glasses when cutting the muscle. After muscle dissection, we can see the layer containing the venous plexus and the mucosa. When this plexus and the mucosa are no longer covered by muscle fibres, the dorsomedian myotomy is complete. Mucosal lesions can be avoided using this technique. The constrictor muscle is pushed to the side bluntly (Step 7). The newly produced muscle attachments are sutured onto the prevertebral musculature 1 cm paramedially (Step 9) (Fig. 3). The defect caused by larynx resection is reconstructed generally by the platysma fascia flap (Step 11). At the end of the operation, the laryngeal muscle stumps are sewn at the flap so that the horseshoe-form of the musculature tract is preserved (Step 15) (Fig. 4). Additionally, myotomy of the circular muscle fibres is also performed (Step 6b) at the entrance of the oesophagus, as described above.

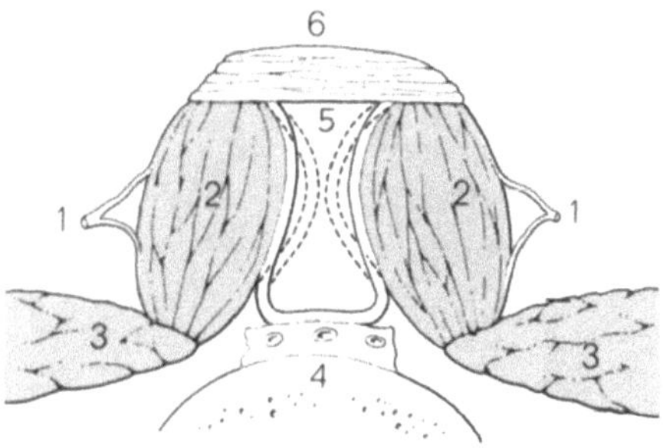

Fig. 4. Functional pharynx surgery. To produce voice the external branch of the cranial laryngeal nerve (*1*) innervates the constrictor muscle (*2*). Good voice modulation depends on the muscle stretch ability

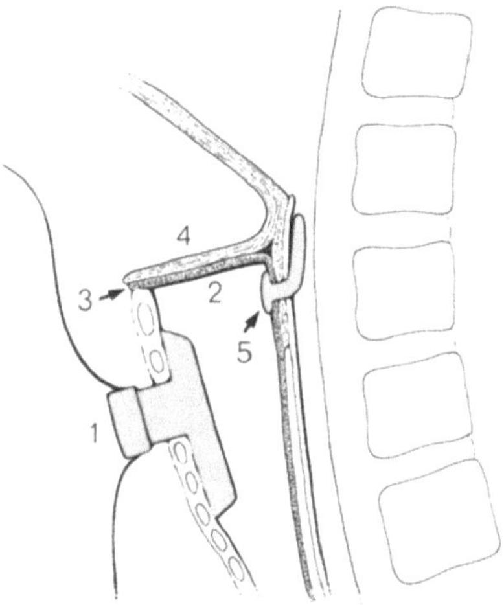

Fig. 5. Tracheostomaplasty and shunt surgery. *1*, The valve stent is inserted in the tracheostoma; *2*, the tracheal chimney; *3*, the roof of the tracheal chimney is closed by the caudally-pediculated mucosal flap of the tracheal dorsal wall; *4*, and by the platysma-fascia-flap; *5*, the shunt is situated on the opposite side of the tracheostoma and strengthened by the platysma-fascia-flap (*4*)

b) Tracheostomaplasty

The tracheostoma is projected onto the anterior trachea wall at the same level as the 3rd and 4th tracheal ring (Fig. 5). 2 intact tracheal rings are preserved above the tracheostoma to form a tracheal chimney. The tracheostoma must be round and should be close to the tracheostoma stent so as to diminish the noise caused by airflow and secretion alongside the tracheostoma valve or finger and to improve voice intelligibility. A standardized tracheostoma helps the patient to seal it tightly and allows a tracheostoma valve insertion. The front third of the 3rd and 4th tracheal cartilage is excised and the mucosa is incised in a cross shape. The skin adhesive silicon stencil is fixed onto the neck skin at the site of the intended tracheostoma (Step 4). The area of the skin to be excised is marked and the skin

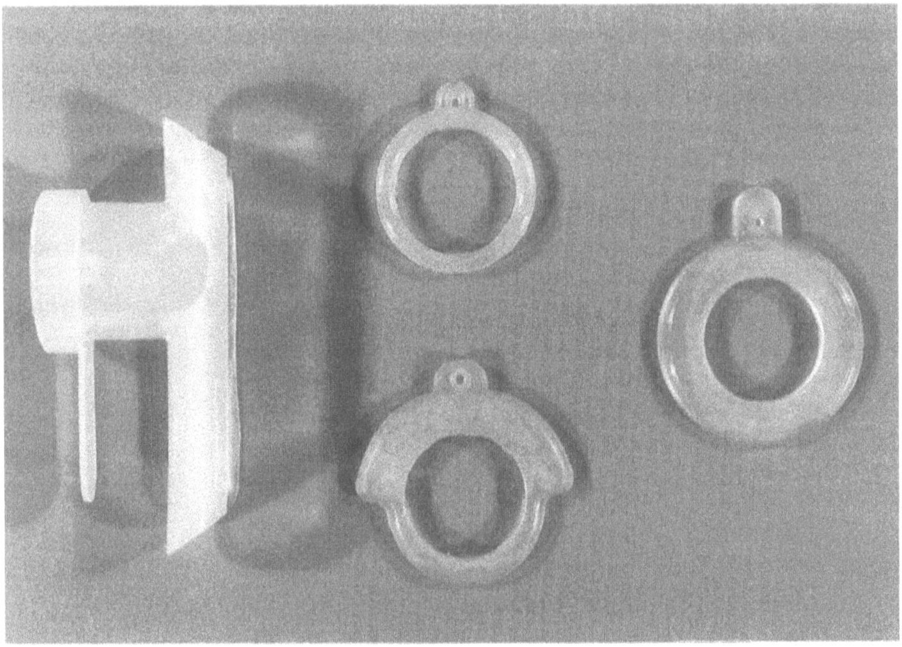

Fig. 6. Tracheostoma valve stent with three different retention collars

is then resected. The suture of skin and mucosa then follows so as to form the tracheostoma (Step 16). The roof of the tracheal chimney is closed by the caudally-pediculated mucosal flap of the tracheal dorsal wall (Step 10). A second covering layer is formed by the platysma-fascia flap (Step 14) or by the pharyngeal mucosa. After the formation of the tracheostoma and glottoplasty with functional pharynx surgery, a tracheostoma stent is inserted (Step 17). Respiration is free from risk (Fig. 6). The technique of tracheostoma stent insertion during surgical treatment was adopted so as to avoid destroying the tracheostomaplasty while changing the tube.

c) Shunt Surgery

We prepare the instrumental set before surgery. For shunt surgery in combination with tracheostomaplasty we use short stents. The end of the puncture needle is moistened with 70% alcohol and is pushed into the open end of the stent. This assembly is then autoclaved for 10 min at 130 °. During this procedure, the silicon of the stent shrinks onto the needle and cannot be displaced during puncture. The needle needs to be sharpened regularly to ensure easy handling. Due to tracheostomaplasty it was necessary to perform the puncture (Step 8). The pharynx itself is spread out. The puncture needle is kept with the handle and is directed outwards through the middle of the digestive tract and the posterior tracheal wall. The outer retention collar is then positioned. The stent and needle are disconnected. The shunt should be situated on the opposite side of the tracheostoma.

One part of the pediculated platysma fascia flap should be interposed in a regular way between the respiratory tract and the digestive tract in order to strengthen the shunt.

It is necessary to strengthen the shunt because the anterior wall of the oesophagus entrance at this point is 2.4 to 2.6 mm thick, which compares with 1.2 to 1.5 mm thickness of the same wall at the end below the 3rd tracheal ring. In 3 cases, the prosthesis shifted in the absence of strengthening and in 2 cases the shunt extended after surgical treatment.

After puncture, the above-mentioned platysma flap is split twice (Step 12) so that one part of the flap protects the tracheal chimney and the other one can strengthen the shunt. The incized platysma flap is sewn around the voice prosthesis stent (Step 13).

Postoperative Care

The tracheostoma valve stent is made of very soft silicon and has to be changed every day. Proper care of the tracheostomaplasty helps to protect against infection and necrosis. Before removal of the dietary tube, the oesophagus is monitored by contrast radiography in order to determine its position and width.

Insertion of the Prosthesis

Normally, the prosthesis is inserted 10 to 12 days postoperatively after the removal of the dietary tube. The position of the digestive tract is properly considered throughout the procedure. During the first few days after prosthesis insertion, phonation may be aggravated by mucous swelling. Swollen tissue may disturb the air flow to open the pharynx. The valve is thus very seldom pressed during deglutition.

Stent Insertion

Should this be needed, the tracheal mucosa is desensitized with a local anaesthetic and the prosthesis extracted. We then insert the stent with the inserter described in the chapter "Hypopharyngeal Puncture" (p. 43). The stent is left in place until the swelling subsides. We use the same procedure to alleviate tissue reaction after radiation therapy.

Prosthesis Change

Normally, these self-cleaning prostheses can be used for several months without any complications. The prosthesis change is described in the chapter "Hypopharyngeal Puncture" (p. 43). When a long prosthesis creates a poor breathing sound, we have to insert a shorter one. If the patient has a short prosthesis which needs a high pressure for voice production, we insert a longer one.

Tracheostoma Valve

The use and technique of the tracheostoma valve is described in a later chapter (p. 184).

Results

We have performed 135 primary voice restorations. The improved primary technique described above was used on 38 patients. Voice quality is confirmed by in vivo measurements of flow resistance and speech analysis. Good voice modulation ability is attained after glottoplasty with functional pharynx surgery and brief speech therapy. Deglutition remains unimpaired.

Reference

Herrmann IF, Koss W (1985) Die fingerfreie Sprache nach totaler Laryngektomie. HNO 33:124–129

Chapter 5 Indications, Results and Their Means of Evaluation

Possible Ways of Reconstructing the Pharynx with a One-Step Operation while Attempting Voice Restoration

I. F. HERRMANN [1]

A laryngectomy is needed in most cases where there are extensive carcinomas of the hypopharynx. Once the partial or total resection of the hypopharynx has been performed it needs to be reconstructed. One-step reconstructions are preferred. In order to be able to determine the extent of change in the mucous membrane during resection and to exclude a possible multi-focal tumor metastasis, o-toluidine blue is applied intraoperatively. If the tumor has spread into the pharynx, or if we are dealing primarily with a hypopharyngeal carcinoma ending not less than 2 cm before the oesophagus orifice, the tumor is resected with 2.5 cm safety zone. For the purposes of surgical voice rehabilitation and satisfactory deglutition, pharynx reconstruction is indicated if the remaining part of the pharynx tube is less than 3 cm wide. Thus, food intake is unimpeded along side the valve prosthesis.

A simultaneous reconstruction of the musculocutaneous flaps, e.g., the major pectoral muscle or the platysma fascia flap (Herrmann) is appropriate in the above cases.

If the tumor has already reached the oeosophageal orifice or if a primary carcinoma of the oesophageal entrance is involved, a laryngectomy and an oesophagectomy is then indicated because of the necessary circular safety zone of 5 cm. In such cases a reconstruction is made with a transmediastinal stomach transposition and an accompanying pharyngogastrostomy.

1. The Musculocutaneous Flap of the Major Pectoral Muscle

Technique (Fig. 1). The hairless skin under the mamilla is best suited for a replacement of the pharynx. In case of total replacement the mamilla must be drawn into the flap. The surgical procedure involving the preparation and preservation of the pectoral ramus of the thoracoacromialis artery as a flap-sustaining vessel is well described in the literature.

Results. 62 musculocutaneous flaps were implanted. 6 partial or total necroses of the flaps were observed. In 29 cases, the flap was used for either the partial or the total replacement of the pharynx. One-third of these patients developed a pharyngeal fistula. This was due to the relatively high rigidity of the flap which alters the

[1] Universitätsklinik und Poliklinik für Hals-, Nasen- und Ohrenkranke im Kopfklinikum, D-8700 Würzburg.

Speech Restoration Via Voice Prostheses
Edited by I. F. Herrmann

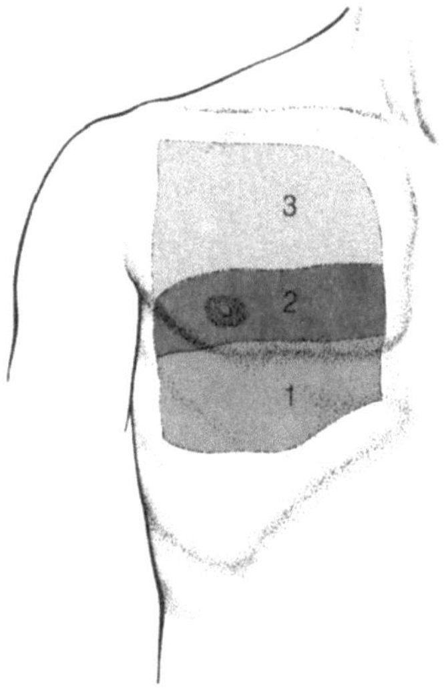

Fig. 1. The hairless skin under the mamilla is best suited for a replacement of the pharynx. *1*, Skin for partial hypopharynx replacement; *1*, *2*, skin for total hypopharynx replacement

shape of the neopharynx tube, especially when there is abundant fatty tissue. This is why we do not fix subcutaneous fatty tissue to the muscle root.

The different tissue types and thicknesses make it difficult to incorporate the flap. One advantage is that there is no shrinkage even after many years as nerve contact is preserved. As a rule, surgical voice rehabilitation is usually performed simultaneously.

2. The Platysma Fascia Flap

Technique. The fascia colli media protects the inner side of the flap between the sternocleidomastoidei muscles. Elsewhere the flap is protected by the outer part of the superficial fascia (Fig. 2). The flap is innervated by the colli ramus of the acial nerve and its blood supply derives from the branches of the facial artery. The flap is pediculated cranially.

Results. Of the 46 flaps we have implanted, only one total necrosis has been observed to date. This was where a patient ate and drank independently of his feeding tube despite our strictest instructions on the second postoperative day. In two other cases, we observed a pharyngeal fistula which spontaneously subsided. In one case, an extensive necrosis of the outer skin occurred which required extensive treatment. Small superficial skin necroses were seen in 8 cases.

Since then, we loosen the skin from the platysma fascia flap only as little as absolutely necessary to guard against any possible defects. One advantage is that the pharynx wall has a similar tissue type and thickness. This facilitates the incorporation of the flap into the pharynx. For total replacements, a silicon stent must be inserted until the flap has been epithelialised in order to avoid stenoses. Surgical voice rehabilitation is usually performed simultaneously.

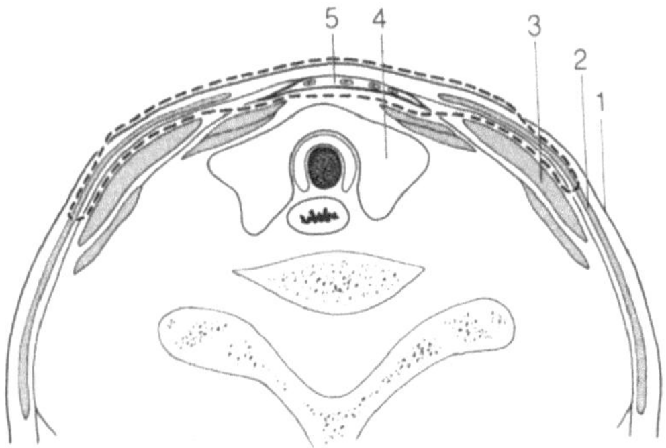

Fig. 2. Scheme for the preparation of the platysma fascia flap. The *broken line* shows the region where the platysma fascia flap is incised. *1*, Skin; *2*, platysma; *3*, sternocleidomastoideus muscle; *4*, thyroid gland; *5*, fascia colli superficialis/vessels/fascia colli media

3. Stomach Transposition with Pharyngogastrostomy and Laterotension of the Stomach

Technique. After the mobilisation of the larynx and the pharynx, the cervical oesophagus is loosened bluntly from the surrounding tissue. Together with the tumor block, the oesophagus is mobilized bluntly and caudally through the upper thorax aperture. The surgeon mobilizes the oesophagus bluntly from the abdomen, removes it, and resects the tumor mass. After the stomach has been mo-

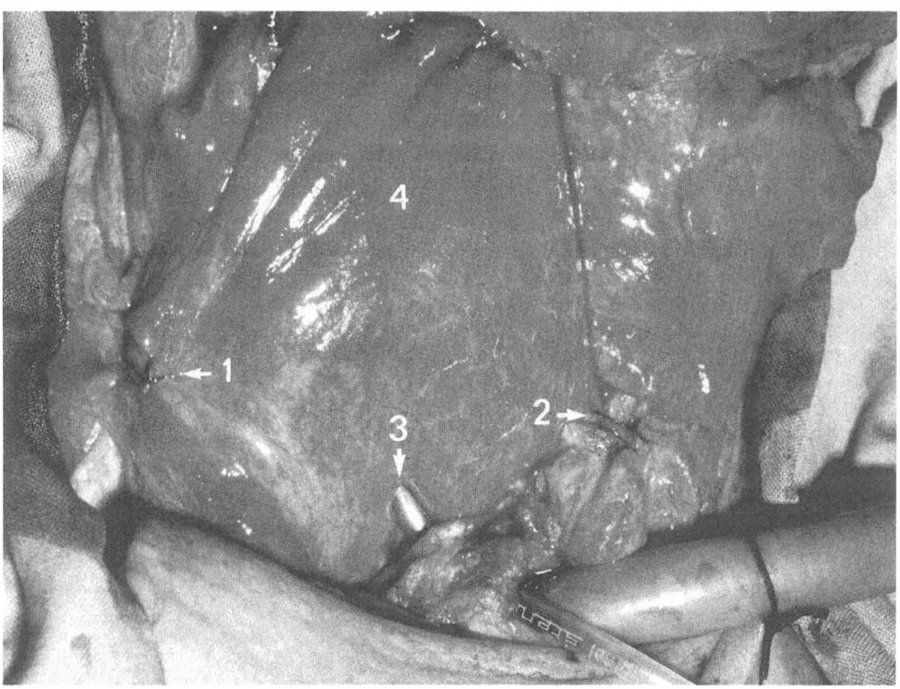

Fig. 3. Laterotension of the stomach. Contact between the walls of the mucous membrane above the shunt guarantees satisfactory voice production. *1*, *2*, Laterotension of the stomach; *3*, shunt with silicone stent; *4*, stomach

bilized while preserving vessel supply, it is then transposed transmediastinally or retrosternally as described by Akiyama (1980) and Ong (1969). After opening the stomach fundus, the pharynx rear and side walls are sutured to the wall of the stomach. Puncture and shunt reinforcement enable surgical voice rehabilitation via the platysmal flap. The stomach is stretched over the shunt by two stitches and sutured to the throat musculature while remaining attached to the pharynx (Fig. 3). Contact between the anterior and posterior wall of the stomach is thus obtained above the valve prosthesis. This guarantees satisfactory voice production once the wound has healed and the voice prosthesis has been inserted.

Results. A total of 16 stomach transpositions were performed after laryngopharyngo-oesophagectomy using glotto plasty (surgical voice rehabilitation). In 3 cases, an anastomosis insufficiency occurred. The operation region had become infected by a tracheotomy which had had to be performed several days before the transposition. Pleural effusion was observed in 4 cases. The average survival period of the patient was only 8 months. 2 patients, however, are recidive-free to this day. Patients' deaths were predominantly due to distant metastases. Preoperative difficulties such as impeded deglutition and respiration were corrected by the operation. Our surgery saves the patient breathing and deglutition difficulties, obstruction and the necessary implant of a feeding fistula, tumor exulceration of the throat, and massive lymphedema in the facial area with macroglossy. Voice was reproduced in every case. Nevertheless, this operation should only be performed in selected cases on account of the surgical risk.

References

Akiyama H (1980) Surgery of carcinoma of the oesophagus – Current problems in surgery. Year Book Medical Publishers, Chicago London

Ariyan S (1982) An analysis of 133 pectoralis major myocutaneous flaps. Plast Reconstr Surg 69:468

Herrmann IF, Buchwald J, Zenner HP (1983) Die Glottoplastik – eine neue Methode zur chirurgischen Stimmrehabilitation. HNO 32:124–129

Herrmann IF (1984) Anmerkungen zur Verwendung des myokutanen Lappens des Musculus pectoralis major. Laryng Rhinol Otol 63:277–282

Herrmann IF (1984) Die Pharynxrekonstruktion mit dem Platysma-Faszienlappen. Laryng Rhinol Otol 63:273–276

Krajina Z, Kosokovic F, Većerina S (1979) Laryngeal reconstruction with sternohyoid fascia in partial laryngectomy. J Laryngol Otol 93:1181

Ong GB (1969) Carcinoma of the hypopharynx and cervical oesophagus. In. Smith R (ed) Progress in clinical surgery, series III. Churchill, London, p 155

Problem of the Indications for the Use of a Valved Prosthesis

E. MOZOLEWSKI and C. TARNOWSKA [1]

The valve prosthesis has not been very frequently used by those patients who were laryngectomized in our Department (about 2 patients per year from 1969 to 1983). The reasons for this are:

1. The development of our own quite successful methods of reconstructive surgery after subtotal laryngectomy and of autoplastic vocal shunts (Mozolewski et al. 1980)
2. Our own plastic surgery on the pharyngo-oesophageal sphincter (Mozolewski et al. 1984) enabling the swift mastery of oesophageal voice in 93% of laryngectomized patients (av. time = 2 weeks, min. 1 day, max. 2 months).

Moreover, the quality of the resultant oesophageal voice has perceptual and acoustic characteristics resembling the laryngeal one (Tarnowska et al. 1984). Taking the above-mentioned possibilities into account, the valve prostheses are only used in patients where there is great surgical risk. Such cases would be after heavy radiation therapy and where there is not sufficient motivation or time to master oesophageal voice. It would seem that any choice between the valve prosthesis or autoplastic shunt and oesophageal voice, disregarding the problem of leakage, depends on the degree of energy consumption during phonation and the perceptual and acoustic characteristics of voice.

References

Mozolewski E et al. (1980) Primary mucoplastic vocal shunt. In: Shedd D, Weinberg B, Hall GK (eds) Surgical and prosthetic approaches to speech rehabilitation. Boston, USA
Mozolewski E et al. (1984) Myotomy with interposition: its technique and results. Otolaryng Pol
Tarnowska C et al. (1984) Esophageal voice following myotomy of pharyngo-oesophageal sphincter. Otolaryng Pol

[1] Ul. Unii Lubelskiej Nr. 1, 71-344 Szczecin, Poland.

Speech Restoration Via Voice Prostheses
Edited by I. F. Herrmann

Lung Function Tests in Laryngectomized Patients

J. BRENDEBACH [1], M. SCHMIDT [2] and E. BRUGGER [2]

1. Introduction

In the literature there are very conflicting views about the cause and extent of the lung function change after laryngectomy. The aim of our investigation was to differentiate between changes in lung function values resulting from the laryngectomy itself and those which occurred because of other accompanying diseases and circumstances (bronchitis, smoking, etc.). Additionally, we intended to find further background data to enable new developments in voice prostheses and tracheostoma valves.

2. Materials and Methods

In our investigation programme, we included all laryngectomized patients who were being treated by the ENT department of Wuerzburg University in 1983. Some of them had already undergone lung function tests in 1981 and some had undergone them before laryngectomy. We had therefore a total number of 115 patients, 30 of whom had been checked both before and after laryngectomy and 24 of whom had been checked twice after operation. The lung function tests had been performed by body-plethysmograph and pneumotachograph.

3. Results

a) Parameter Distribution

We checked 30 parameters in each patient. When measuring the lung function parameters in "% predicted" (using the standards published by the European Community for Coal and Steel), we found that the following parameters were approximately normally distributed: age, weight, and height of patients, vital capacity (VC), forced expiratory volume in 1 s (FEV 1), intrathoracic gas volume (ITGV), residual volume (RV), total lung capacity (TC), peak expiratory flow (PEF), maximum expiratory flow with 50% or 25% remaining VC in the lungs (MEF

[1] Universitätsklinik und Poliklinik für Hals-, Nasen- und Ohrenkranke im Kopfklinikum, D-8700 Würzburg.
[2] Universitätsklinik für Innere Medizin, D-8700 Würzburg.

Speech Restoration Via Voice Prostheses
Edited by I. F. Herrmann

50/25%). The data deviated more than normally for total and expiratory airway resistance [R (kPa/l/s)] and "time after operation" (=time difference between laryngectomy and lung function test).

b) **Cluster Analysis** (Fig. 1)

A cluster analysis showed that a lot of parameters were interrelated. Hence VC corresponded very closely to FEV 1, PEF, and MEF 50/25%, and ITGV very closely to RV and TC. Some results are of special interest:

R as well as the peak inspiratory and expiratory flows in normal (unforced) ventilation ("*IN FLOW*" and "*OUT FLOW*") corresponded more to age, weight, and height than they did to ITGV and VC (Fig. 1).

Conclusion: Only a small number of parameters are needed to measure the lung function of laryngectomized patients. VC and R seemed to be the most important and representative parameters.

c) **Means and Variances** (Table 1)

VC and FEV 1 were on average 30%–40% smaller, and ITGV 30%–40% greater than the standard values. R values showed a wide deviation.

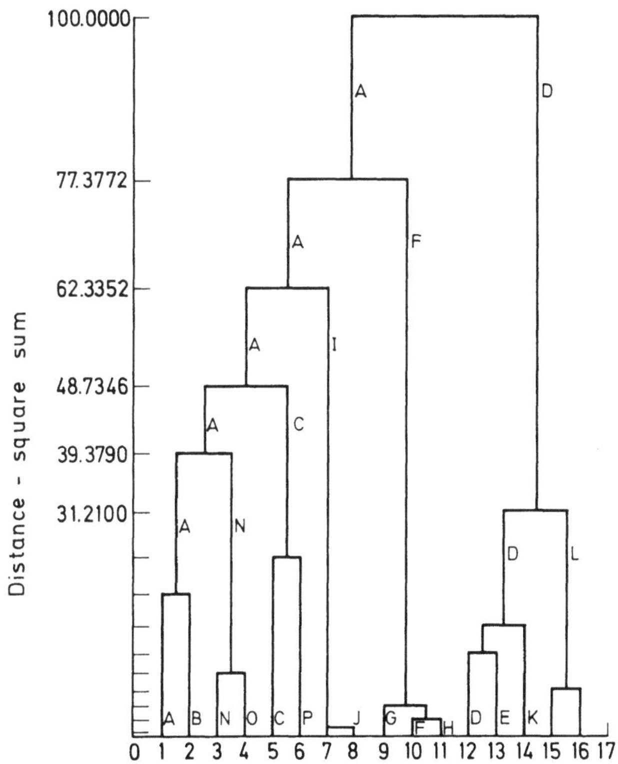

Fig. 1. Cluster analysis. Parameters: *A*, height; *B*, weight; *C*, age; *D*, VC; *E*, FEV 1; *F*, ITGV; *G*, TC; *H*, RV; *I*, R (exp.); *J*, TR (total); *K*, PEF; *L*, MEF 50%; *M*, MEF 25%; *N*, IN FLOW; *O*, OUT FLOW; *P*, time after operation

Table 1. Mean values, standard deviations, and intervals (115 patients)

Parameter	Unit	Mean	Variance	Interval
Age	Years	60.4	10.0	39 – 78
Weight	kg	74.4	11.9	52 –108
Length	cm	170	6.7	158 –188
VC	% pred.	69.2	15.4	30.4 –126.1
FEV 1	% pred.	64.2	19.0	23.9 –122.5
ITGV	% pred.	137.0	30.6	73.9 –273.3
R (total)	kPa/l/s	0.35	0.13	0.07– 1.11

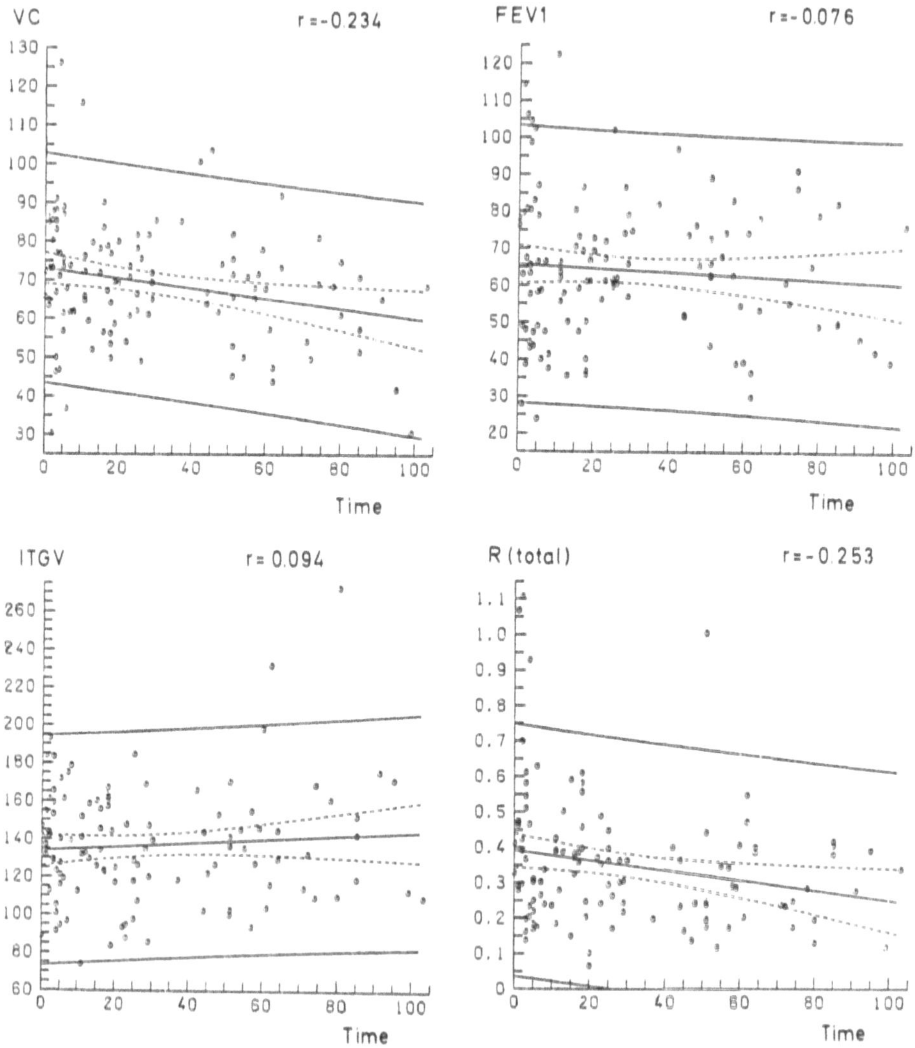

Fig. 2. VC (% pred.), FEV 1 (% pred.), ITGV 1 (% pred.), and R (total) (kPa/1/s) during the "time after operation"

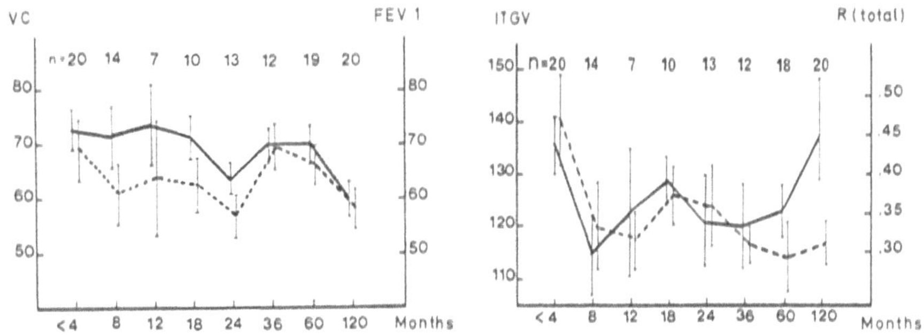

Fig. 3. VC, FEV 1, ITGV, and R in groups according to "time after operation"

d) Correlations (Figs. 2, 3)

In testing the correlation between the parameters, we were mainly interested in how lung function parameters changed against time. We found that VC (% pred.) and P (kPa/l/s) did not decrease significantly whereas FEV 1 (% pred.) and ITGV (% pred.) remained almost static during the "time after operation" (Fig. 2).

When we investigated this problem in more detail by dividing patients into groups according to "time after operation", we found that there was no uniform lung function decrease or increase against time. There were also no significant differences between the groups (Fig. 3).

e) The 24 Patients Who Underwent Two Post-Operative Tests (Table 2)

VC, FEV 1 and ITGV remained rather static whereas R values showed both greater changes and a wide variance.

f) 30 Patients Who Had Undergone Tests Both Before and After the Operation (Table 3)

We observed a decrease in VC, FEV 1 and ITGV from "before" to "after operation" values. This applied to both the mean values and the majority of patients. We found no uniform change in R but a very wide variance of more than 50%. By contrast, standard deviations of VC, FEV 1, and ITGV were less than 20%.

Table 2. Two tests after operation (24 patients)

Parameter	Unit	Mean		Number of patients		
		1. Test	2. Test	Increase	Decrease	Change <20%
VC	% pred.	66.7	66.4	11	13	20
FEV 1	% pred.	63.1	61.5	10	14	11
ITGV	% pred.	125.3	122.3	18	6	19
R (total)	kPa/l/s	0.45	0.33	18	6	3

Table 3. Tests before and after operation (30 patients)

Parameter	Unit	Mean		Number of patients		
		Before	After	Increase	Decrease	Change <20%
VC	% pred.	77.4	67.2	7	23	15
FEV 1	% pred.	73.0	61.0	7	23	11
ITGV	% pred.	148.8	131.1	4	26	18
R (total)	kPa/l/s	0.38	0.36	14	16	5

Discussion

In general, lung function parameters did not decrease or increase significantly more in laryngectomized patients than in healthy people. In contrast to some authors, we believe that lung function parameters are not primarily influenced by the laryngectomy but rather depend on the patient's general situation. The life quality of laryngectomized patients does not seem to be mainly impaired by lung function. We therefore see nor reason why patients should be excluded from voice restoration attempts because of bad lung function parameters alone.

References

Blechschmidt M, de l'Espine Th, Brugger E, Herrmann IF (1982) Untersuchung der Korrelation zwischen Lungenfunktion und Stimmverhalten nach Glottoplastik. Laryng Rhinol Otol 61:261

Fouarge M (1964) Etude des problèmes respiratoires avant et après laryngectomie. Acta Oto-Rhino-Laryng Belg 18:579–600

Giesen M, Dorow P (1978) Die Auswirkung der Laryngektomie auf die Lungenfunktion. Arch ORL (Berlin) 219:390–391

Herrmann IF (to be published) Experiences with the ESKA-Herrmann tracheostoma valve in speech restoration via valve prostheses. Springer, Berlin Heidelberg New York Tokyo

Schwab W et al. (1958) Die Lungenfunktion beim Kehlkopflosen. Hüthig, Heidelberg Frankfurt

Togawa K et al. (1980) A physiologic study on respiratory handicap of the laryngectomized. Arch ORL (Berlin) 229:69–79

Evaluation of Speech With and Without a "Groningen Type" Voice Button

H. K. Schutte, E. F. M. Bors, G. H. A de Boer, G. L. J. Nieboer
and A. A. Annyas [1]

Button-assisted oesophageal speech depends on the aerodynamic characteristics of the button itself and on its physiological consequences. The valve part of the button must prevent leakage into the trachea. On the other hand, air must pass as easily as possible from the trachea into the oesophagus. Air from the lungs must be directed into the oesophagus. This is done either by closing the patient's tracheostoma with fingers or thumb or by a specially-designed automatic tracheostoma valve.

The physiological background of button-assisted oesophageal voice production is very different from the popular injection oesophageal voice production method. Injection oesophageal voice, for which a training method was developed by Moolenaar-Bijl at Groningen in the early fifties, uses the injection of small amounts of air into the oesophagus together with explosive consonants in normal speech. In 1953 the physiological background was clarified by van den Berg and Damsté (1958). In button-assisted oesophageal speech, the required increase in air pressure below the neoglottis, which vibrates the neoglottis, is easily achieved by a continuous airway connection between the trachea and a small air chamber below the neoglottis. This pressure chamber, from which air escapes through the neoglottis, is constantly refilled by a continuous stream of air from the lungs. In contrast to the injection method, the amount of air which can be used for ongoing phonation by using a button is much larger. In button-assisted oesophageal speech, moreover, the air pressure below the neoglottis can be controlled by the same muscular mechanisms as with normal laryngeal voice production. Of course, differences between laryngeal speech and button-assisted oesophageal voice production exist especially as far as the height of the air pressure is concerned. These pressure differences are partly explained by the driving pressure needed to maintain vibration of the tissue structures in the oesophageal neoglottis and partly by the pressure needed to overcome the resistance of the button itself. These aspects are discussed in greater detail by Nieboer (1985). The differences in physiological background, e.g., the better air control, seem to explain the greater vocal possibilities which are generally found in patients with a button. The different physiological factors have important consequences for the training of the laryngectomees as well as for the quality of the artificial voice. The differences between the training programmes for injection oesophageal voice and button-assisted oesophageal voice are explained by Bors (1984).

[1] University Hospital Groningen, 9700 RB Groningen, The Netherlands.

Speech Restoration Via Voice Prostheses
Edited by I. F. Herrmann

We will confine ourselves in this paper to our standardized evaluation programme for both types of oesophageal voice substitute. For a proper evaluation of our rehabilitation results, it does not seem correct to compare button-assisted oesophageal voice with injection oesophageal voice without considering the differences in voice production possibilities.

In order to compare the speech performance of oesophageal voice for both types, we developed criteria that would differentiate them both. The final judgement is based upon a weighted evaluation of three Main Criteria Groups:

1. Phonatory Skills
2. Additional factors, and
3. the overall subjective opinion of the researcher.

For each Main Criteria Group a three point scale was used: Good, Moderate, and Poor. The criteria used, were based on the speech performance data of the first 17 of our patients to use button-assisted oesophageal voice. From this, it can be concluded that the vocal performance of button-assisted speech differed strikingly in at least four aspects from injection oesophageal voice. Data for injection oesophageal voice were taken from the literature and appeared to be practically the same as found in our clinic. The criteria used for objective measurable data of the first Main Criteria Group are given in Table 1. This shows how we defined the evaluations: Good, Moderate and Poor for each oesophageal voice type. The differentiations were established by obtaining the values of our 5 best and 5 worst button speakers.

Up to 19 syllables were needed to achieve "good" button voice. Below nine syllables was considered "poor". This contrasts strikingly with injection oesophageal voice where more than 5 syllables per injection are considered "good". The same applies for the other aspects mentioned above. What we call "good" for injection oesophageal voice is considered "poor" for button-assisted oesophageal voice. The maximum sound pressure level which can be reached by button-assisted oesophageal voice also appeared to be higher than with injection oesophageal voice. One of our best button speakers could reach 95 dB 30 cm from the

Table 1. Criteria for objective measurable data of phonatory skills

		Button	Injection
a) Syllables per intake of air	Good	≧19	≧ 5
	Moderate	10–18	2 –4
	Poor	≦ 9	1
b) Max. phonation time in seconds	Good	≧10	≧ 2
	Moderate	4– 9	0.5–2
	Poor	≦ 3	≦ 0.5
c) Dynamic Range in dB	Good	≧25	>20 dB is rare
	Moderate	16–24	
	Poor	≦15	
d) Max. S.P.L. (30 cm dB (A))	Mean	78 dB	>70 dB is rare
	Range	65–95 dB	

Table 2. Success rate of substitute oesophageal voice: Percentages "good +moderate" = useful oesophageal voice with a weighted evaluation of button-assisted and injection oesophageal voice

	Patients without button	Patients with button		
	Injection n=49	Injection	Button	
1 week	47 (12+35)	50 (25+25)	65 (54+11)	n=35
1 months	65 (12+53)	63 (29+34)	79 (62+17)	
3 months	78 (43+35)	60 (31+29)	78 (62+16)	
6 months	82 (45+37)	73 (27+46)	95 (86+ 9)	n=13
12 months	83 (55+28)	59 (36+23)	86 (81+ 5)	

microphone. This means that a button speaker is able to produce intelligible speech in a noisy environment.

Other phonatory skill aspects such as availability, voice pitch modulation, articulation, speech rate, and speech fluency are also favored by using button-assisted oesophageal voice. These skills determine a patient's overall communicative potential to a great extent. Speaking is more natural when using a button. The above-mentioned aspects have to be judged more subjectively because of the lack of clear parameters which are suited to clinical settings. We also use a three point scale for evaluation purposes as with the other two Main Criteria Group. This time, we evaluate the audibility of stoma noise and other noises connected with the dexterity of stoma closure in button patients. In patients with injection oesophageal voice, we evaluate both audible stoma noise and any extra movements of the head and mouth when speaking.

The final judgment is also made on a three point scale: Good, Moderate and Poor. For this we summarize our measured and given evaluations in the 3 Main Criteria Groups according to certain set rules. Substitute oesophageal voice is called "good" if no more than 3 evaluations of "moderate" are recorded in the Main Criteria Groups I and II; the resting ratings have to be "good". A "moderate" rating is given if no more than one aspect was considered "poor" in one of the Main Criteria Groups I and II. If an evaluation of "poor" was made twice in any one group or more than 3 times in all, the final rating of the substitute voice is considered "poor".

We used this method to evaluate the speech results of patients with and without button. We also evaluated the injection oesophageal voice in patients with a button. Evaluations were made at fixed intervals after the start of the rehabilitation: after 1 week and after 1, 3, 6, and 12 months. The results are given in Table 2.

We examined 49 patients without a button and 35 patients with a button. In the left-hand column, the data of injection oesophageal voice in patients without a button are given. The middle column gives the results of injection oesophageal voice in patients who have a button. The right-hand column shows the data of button-assisted oesophageal speech. The figures represent the sum of "good" and "moderate" scores which are given separately in brackets.

The success rate of useful oesophageal speech is up to 85% for injection oesophageal voice as well as for button-assisted oesophageal voice. Whilst bearing in mind that higher standards were set for button-assisted oesophageal voice, useful oesophageal speech was attained in 85% of cases. A "good" rating was still given in 81% of button-assisted oesophageal speech. In patients with injection oesophageal voice without a button, only 55% of voices were found to be "good". This again supports the superiority of button-assisted oesophageal voice.

A more precise analysis of the "good" and "moderate" scores reveals that only 12% of patients without a button attain good injection oesophageal speech after 1 week. In patients with a button, the percentage of patients attaining good injection oesophageal speech after 1 week is as high as 25%. Moreover, good button-assisted oesophageal speech could be found in more than 50% of cases after 1 week. This is very important for rehabilitation purposes because most of our patients are able to make themselves clearly understood with a good substitute voice as soon as they leave hospital. This also means that they regain their voice 2.5 weeks after the operation and after 1 week of therapy.

From our investigations we concluded that button-assisted oesophageal speech enables much better phonatory skills. This forced us to develop new criteria for comparisons with injection oesophageal voice. It can also be seen from the data that button placement during laryngectomy provides patients with the best chance of successful and fast rehabilitation. Furthermore, we have established that patients prefer to use injection oesophageal voice after a while for 2 reasons: firstly, the quality of injection oesophageal voice improves in time, and secondly, many patients feel hampered in their social life when they have to use one hand for speaking. Further development of a practical automatic stoma valve would therefore seem to be very necessary indeed.

Nevertheless, we still advocate the application of a button because voice rehabilitation during the first weeks after laryngectomy is much easier to achieve.

References

Berg van den Jw et al. (1958) Oesophageal speech. Folia Phoniatrica 10:65–84

Bors EFM et al. (1984) Speech training of oesophageal voice by using a button. Proceedings XIX Congr of the IALP, Vol III:937–941

Damsté PH (1958) Oesophageal speech after laryngectomy. Dissertation, Groningen

Moolenaar-Bijl AJ (1953) The importance of certain consonants in oesophageal voice after laryngectomy. Ann Otol Rhinol Laryngol 62:979–989

Nieboer GLJ, Schutte HK (1985) Aerodynamical properties of buttons and of button assisted oesophageal speech. In: Speech Restoration via Voice Prostheses. Int. Workhop June 1984, Würzburg

Intelligibility, Vocal Intensity, and Long-Term Average Spectra of Groningen Button-Oesophageal Speech

H. F. MAHIEU, H. K. SCHUTTE and A. A. ANNYAS[1]

Introduction

Most, if not all, of my colleagues who have any experience of tracheo-oesophageal fistula speech production, agree that this type of voice production is louder, more fluent, and more intelligible than other methods of speech production available to laryngectomees. This widely held opinion is primarily based on subjective observations and cannot evaluate the voice qualities of the different voice production types objectively. We all think that tracheo-oesophageal fistula voice production, or button-assisted oesophageal speech as we prefer to call it, is superior to conventional oesophageal speech. Little or no effort, however, has been made to research effectively the differences between the various voice production methods by measuring such parameters as volume, intelligibility, and fluency. If we want to compare speech quality results, it is essential to use standardized measurements.

The aim of our study was to compare the vocal communication ability of the button method laryngectomee with the conventional injection method laryngectomee and further to compare both these methods with normal laryngeal speech. To do this, we employed several perceptual and acoustic measuring methods. One of these methods is the speech penetration capacity (SPC) test which determines the intelligibility of speech in a noisy environment regardless of the intensity level of the speech produced. In other words, to what extent can a speaker make himself understood in a noisy environment without having to raise his voice? This mainly depends on two factors:

- How loudly can he speak?
- What is the penetrating capacity of his speech in a noisy environment?

Besides the SPC, it was therefore also necessary to measure maxium vocal intensity while speaking loudly and while shouting as loud as possible across a room, which we shall refer to hereafter as calling. These measurements seemed a good way of determining the vocal communication abilities of our patients.

It is only to be expected that differences in SPC are connected with spectral components in produced speech signals. Therefore, it was decided to measure the long-term average spectra (LTAS) of a spoken text. It is obvious that objective measurements are needed to determine the quality of button-assisted oesophageal voice production. Care, however, must be used when comparing data from conventional oesophageal speech. This is because of the differences in the underlying

[1] Academic Hospital Groningen, 9700 RB Groningen, The Netherlands.

Speech Restoration Via Voice Prostheses
Edited by I. F. Herrmann

physiological mechanisms between the button method and the injection method of speech production (Schutte et al. 1985). Standards of successful conventional oesophageal speech also vary greatly according to various criteria, e.g., the country and medical centre where the patient attends his speech rehabilitation programme. Our clinic has a tradition in injection oesophageal speech training. This may be one of the reasons for the fact that 85% of all our laryngectomized patients acquire good to moderate injection oesophageal speech (Schutte et al. 1985).

Successful oesophageal speech patients in the United States do not usually exceed 50% (Schaeffer and Johns 1982; Gates et al. 1982). The high successrate of our injection oesophageal speech course sets a high standard of comparison for button-assisted oesophageal speech.

Materials and Methods

31 laryngectomized patients, who all received the Groningen button, participated in this study. There were 29 males and 2 females with a mean age of almost 61 years (range 38 years to 76 years). All patients were initially trained in both speech methods. No selection criteria were used other than that the Groningen button had to be in place for at least 4 months. 4 of these patients no longer used the button while speaking. 17 of the 31 patients were able to speak with the injection method as well as with the button method of speech, which made them useful for the purposes of comparison. Furthermore, 20 normal laryngeal speakers, 15 males and 5 females, with a mean age of almost 24 years (range 21 years to 27 years) served as a reference.

The SPC-score was determined by letting the subject read aloud 50 words of a Dutch phoneme-balanced wordlist with the injection speech method, and another 50 words from the same list with the button speech method. Normal laryngeal speakers read 100 words aloud from the same list. A tape recording was made of the subject reading the list. This tape recording is later presented to the same subject by means of headphones through which an interfering cocktail party-type noise is added. The sound pressure level of this background noise can be raised in steps of 5 decibels. It is therefore possible to interpolate the noise level so that the subject can understand 50% of the recorded list. The average sound pressure level of the tape recording can be measured and subtracted from the determined noise level resulting in the SPC-score:

dB N − db W = SPC

dB N = the average sound pressure level of the interfering noise (in dB)

dB W = the average sound pressure level of the wordlist recorded (in dB).

A positive SPC-score means that although the noise is louder than the spoken text, the subject can still understand 50%. A negative SPC-score signifies that at the same level of 50% intelligibility, the noise is quieter than the spoken text. Some patients were not able to achieve the 50% intelligibility level for one or either methods, even when no interfering noise was used. This is signified by $-\infty$ and for averaging purposes the result of minus 25 decibels is used in these cases.

The maximum vocal intensity level of speech was measured while speaking loudly and while calling. The subject-to-microphone distance was 1 meter. The test person puts on headphones and is requested to read a text aloud at a level which he/she can just hear. If he/she cannot be heard, then he/she is instructed to read as loudly as possible. While reading the text, the same interfering noise comes through the headphones as in the SPC test with an intensity level increasing up to 90 dB. At a certain point, the subject will no longer hear his own speech and attain his maximum speaking level which can then be registered simply. The maximum vocal intensity during calling is determined by asking the subject to call out the following as loudly as possible: "Hey, you, telephone!"

For the long term average spectral analysis (LTAS), a tape recording is made of each subject reading a short text aloud in Dutch with a duration of about 1 minute at normal reading-pace. A frequency analysis was made of the running speech with a Princeton applied research FFT real time spectrum analyzer (Model 4512). The resulting graphs are visually compared. In this paper, we only give a few examples of LTAS analysis in the form of preliminary results.

Results

Since our primary concern in this paper is to compare the injection method and the button method of voice production, the 17 patients who were able to use both methods are of special interest. After considering the results in this group, we will give the results of the remaining group of 14 patients, who were not able to use either method of voice production.

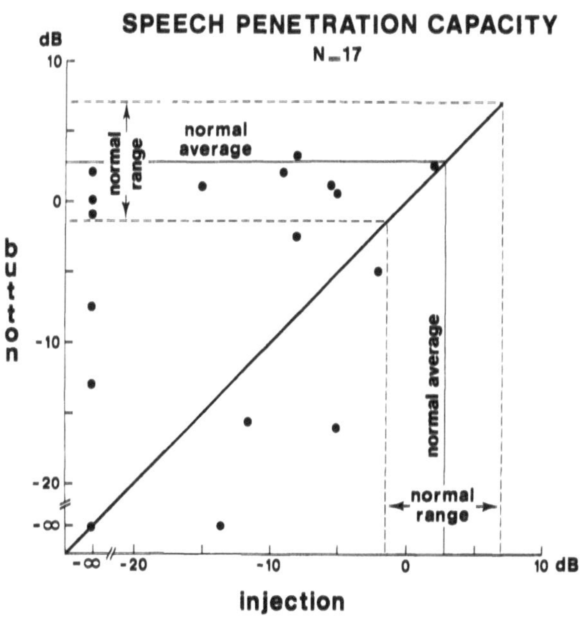

Fig. 1. SPC results of 17 patients able to use both methods of speech. The SPC results for the injection method are given on the horizontal axis. The vertical axis shows the SPC result using the button method of speech. The range and average of the SPC scores of 20 laryngeal speakers serve as a reference (normal range and normal average). For further explanation see text

The results of the SPC test for the 17 patients who were able to use both methods of voice production are given in Fig. 1. The horizontal axis represents the results of the SPC test for the injection method in dBs. The vertical axis shows the results during the button method of voice production. The oblique line in the diagramme is the line where the SPC data of the injection and button methods are equal. Points below this line represent patients with a higher SPC-score when using the injection method, while points above this line represent patients with a higher SPC-score when using the button method of speech. The SPC-scores of the 20 test persons with normal laryngeal voice production serve as reference data and range from −1.5 dB to +7 dB. This range is represented by broken lines in the diagramme (*normal range*). The average reference SPC-score is +2.9 dB and is marked by a continuous line (*normal average*).

12 of the 17 patients have a higher SPC-score when using the button method of voice production, and 9 of these 12 patients are within the normal range when using the button method. The SPC-score of only 1 patient is within the normal range when using the injection method, and even then his button SPC-score is slightly higher. Of the 4 patients who had a higher SPC-score when using the injection method, 3 had not used the button method for at least 4 months before the test. The fourth and best of these patients still preferred the button method because he could then phonate much more loudly and was therefore considered more intelligible when using the button method. The average SPC-score for the patient group with the button method was −5.8 dB, and the average SPC-score for the same group with the injection method was −13.5 dB.

Figure 2 shows maximum vocal intensity results while speaking loudly for 15 patients who were able to use both methods. We were unable to obtain these data for the other 2 patients who could speak with both methods. Both were patients

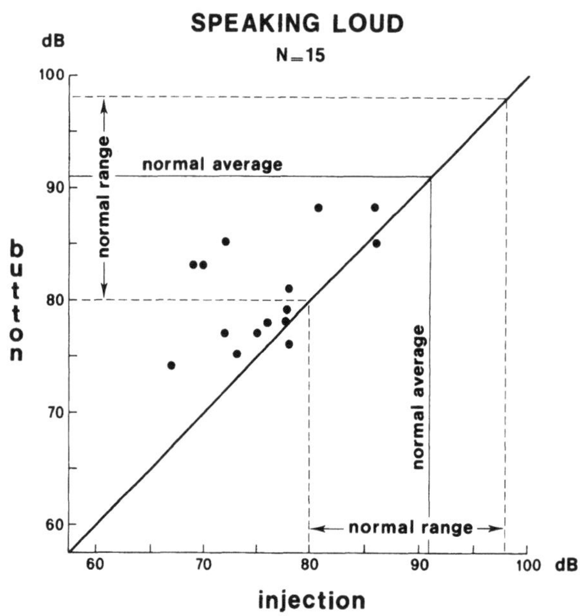

Fig. 2. Results of maxium intensity while speaking loudly for 15 patients able to use both methods of voice production. The horizontal axis shows the results using the injection-method. The vertical axis gives the results using the button method. Range and average of maximum vocal intensity results while speaking loudly for 20 laryngeal speakers serve as a reference (normal range and normal average)

who had a higher SPC-score when using the injection speech method. We were able to measure the maximum vocal intensity while calling for 1 of these patients. He was able to call more loudly when using the button speech method. In Fig. 2, the results of the injection method are given on the horizontal axis, whereas the results of the button method are given on the vertical axis. The average maximum vocal intensity of normal laryngeal speakers while speaking loudly is 91.2 dB (*normal average*) with a range of 80 dB–98 dB (*normal range*). This is represented in Fig. 2 in the same way as in Fig. 1. The oblique line represents where the maximum vocal intensity of the button and injection method are equal. 13 of the 15 patients were able to speak more loudly when using the button method. Of the 2 patients who spoke more loudly with the injection method, the worst one had not used the button method for 4 months. The results of 7 patients using the button method are within the normal range. This compares with the results of only 3 patients using the injection method. Even then, 2 of these 3 patients spoke more loudly when using the button method. The average maximum vocal intensity of the 15 patients while speaking with the button method was 80.5 dB, whereas the average maximum vocal intensity when speaking with the injection method was 75.9 dB.

In Fig. 3, the results of maximum vocal intensity while calling are given. The average of the reference group of laryngeal speakers is 107.6 dB with a range of

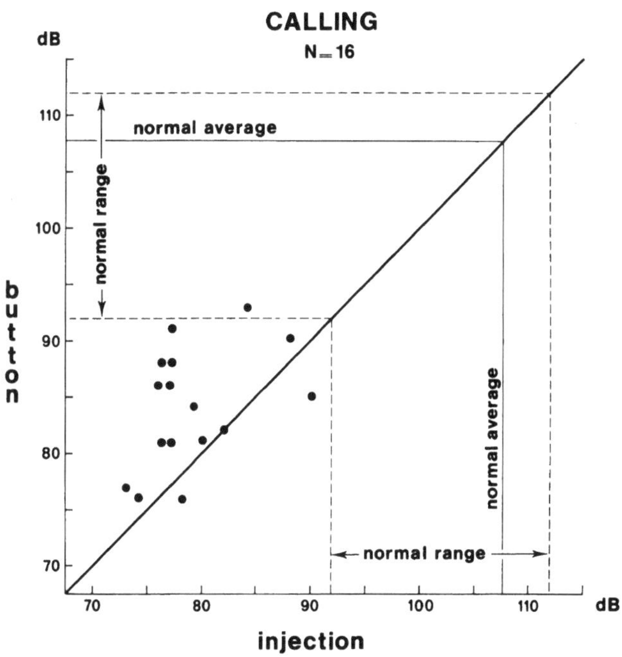

Fig. 3. Results of maximum vocal intensity while calling across a room for 16 patients able to use both voice production methods. The horizontal axis shows the results using the injection method. The vertical axis gives the results using the button method. The range and average of maximum vocal intensity results while calling for 20 laryngeal speakers serve as a reference (normal range and normal average)

92–112 dB (*normal average and normal range*). Only the score of one of the 16 patients is just within the normal range. 13 of these 16 patients called more loudly with the button method than with the injection method. The average maximum vocal intensity when calling with the button method in this group of 16 patients was 84.1 dB, whereas the average maximum vocal intensity when calling with the injection method was 79.2 dB. It is clear that the laryngectomees cannot compete with the normal group as far as vocal intensity during calling is concerned.

Now the results will be given for the remaining group of 14 patients. 13 of them could only speak with the button method (*button speakers*) and 1 of them could onyl use the injection method of voice production (*injection speaker*).

- Only 4 of the 13 button speakers were able to reach a 50% intelligibility level in the SPC-test and only 1 of them was within the normal range. The injection speaker appeared unable to reach the 50% intelligibility level.
- 8 of the 13 button speakers reached a maximum intensity level while speaking loudly which was within the normal range. The average maximum intensity speech level for these 13 patients was 81.1 dB.
- 2 of the 13 button speakers reached a maximum intensity while calling which was within the normal range. The average maximum intensity level of calling for these 13 patients was 85.1 dB.
- The injection speaker reached a maximum intensity of 78 dB while speaking loudly which was also his maximum intensity level while calling.

As has already been mentioned, only a few examples of LTAS analysis can be given here in the form of preliminary results. Figure 4 shows 5 spectrograms. On the horizontal axis the frequency is given in kilocycles (kilohertz), and the vertical axis shows a relative intensity scale in decibels. The first spectrogram is of a normal laryngeal speaker and serves as a reference. The second and third spectrograms are from patient H.: In the second one with the button method and in the third one with the injection method. Patient H. is perceptually judged to be an excellent button speaker but a poor injection oesophageal one. His button SPC-score was +2 dB, whereas his injection SPC-score was $-\infty$ dB (i.e., he could not reach the 50% intelligibility level). His maximum vocal intensity during button method speech was 78 dB and 76 dB with the injection method. During calling these values were 86 dB with the button method and 76 dB with the injection method. His button-speech spectrogram (No. 2) is similar to the normal spectrogram (No. 1), especially in the first formant region below 1 kHz, which is thought to be of major importance. In this patient's injection-speech spectrogram (No. 3), however, the spectrum is rather flat. It stands to reason that this type of speech would hardly be understood in a noisy environment because the first formant is weak and the speech will therefore be totally drowned by only a moderate noise level.

The final 2 spectrograms are from patient B., who is considered to be a good speaker with both methods. He is one of the few patients to have a better injection SPC-score (−2 dB) than a button SPC-score (−4.5 dB). In a noisy environment, however, this patient, favors the button speech method because he is then more readily intelligible with the louder voice of the button method. His maximum vocal intensity with the button method was 83 dB, compared to 69 dB with the injection method. The patient's button-speech spectrogram (No. 4) and injection-

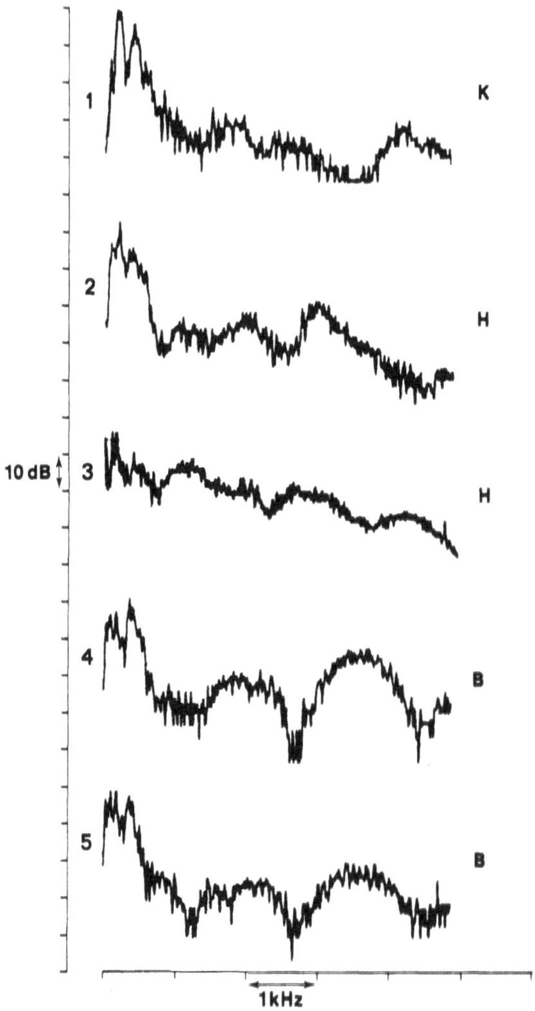

Fig. 4. Long-term average spectrograms. On the horizontal axis the frequency is given from 0–5 kHz. The vertical axis shows a relative intensity scale in dB: *1*, Normal laryngeal speaker K. *2*, Patient H. using the button method (excellent button speaker). *3*, The same patient H. using the injection method (poor injection speaker). *4*, Patient B. using the button method (good button speaker). *5*, The same patient B. using the injection method (good injection speaker)

speech spectrogram (No. 5) have descending slopes comparable with the normal spectrogram. However, the overall slope is slightly steeper in the patient's injection-speech spectrogram. When compared with the button-speech spectrogram (No. 2) of the excellent button speaker H., both spectrograms of patient B., however, show a smaller descending slope.

Discussion of Results

The 17 patients who were able to use both methods of speech were of special interest. This was because we were able to compare the button-assisted oesophageal speech of a patient with his injection oesophageal speech. This eliminated any individual influences on our results such as age, interest, concentration, intelligence, hearingloss (to a moderate extent), etc. In general, it can be stated that not only can most laryngectomees speak more loudly with the button method, but also that their SPC-score is much higher. This meant that their speech has greater intelligibility in a noisy environment. This can be illustrated by comparing the sum of the average SPC-test results and the vocal intensity measurements during speech.

dB SPC + dB max S = max N L

dB max S = the average maximum vocal intensity during speech.

dB SPC = the average SPC

max N L = the average maximum noise load.

This maximum noise load indicates the maximum noise level at which the patient can just make himself understood.

For the injection speech method, this gives:

−13.5 dB + 75.9 dB = 62.4 dB max · noise load.

For the button speech method, this gives:

−5.8 dB + 80.5 dB = 74.4 dB max · noise load.

Normal laryngeal speakers had an average maximum noise load of 2.9 dB + 91.2 dB = 94.2 dB.

The mean difference of about 12 dB in favor of the button method speaker may not seem spectacular. However, if one remembers that a crowded shop or street has a noise level of 65–70 dB, it is easy to see why patients consider the button speech method of a great help in their resocialization process. When comparing these results with those of the reference group, it is obvious that although the button speech method provides greater intelligibility in a noisy environment than the injection speech method, it is still inferior to normal speech. Nonetheless, one of the best button speakers, patient R., who is considered by those who do not know him to be only hoarse or to have a common cold, can attain near normal speech levels with a maximum noise load of 3 dB + 88 dB = 91 dB.

If the results of the group of 14 patients, who were only able to use one method of voice production, are compared with the results of the group of 17 patients who could use both methods, it is obvious that the latter group contains better speakers who have a button speech which is more intelligible in a noisy environment. This finding has been confirmed by trained speech pathologists. This greater intelligibility must be due to a better SPC as there would seem to be no difference between the two patient groups regarding average maximum vocal intensity.

The supremacy of the button method over the injection speech method can also be seen in the preliminary LTAS analysis results which suggest the existence of a correlation between the results of the SPC-test and the descending slope in the spectrogram. LTAS analysis may well be one of the major keys to the objective measurements of speech quality and may clarify the differences in speech intelligibility.

General Discussion

The SPC-test is simple to perform and its results provide a reliable measure of speech intelligibility, which, in combination with the maximum vocal intensity measuring method, can give a good estimation of the subject's vocal communication ability. In the practical SPC-test situation, it is important to consider the patient's hearing acuity. If a patient has severe hearing loss, it may be necessary for an untrained listener with normal hearing to take the listener's place in the test.

Hopefully, LTAS measurements will render more information in the near future on speech intelligibility and the relative importance of the various speech signal elements. We hope that joint efforts will lead to a situation where we can accurately and effectively compare speech results of patient groups from different medical centres. It is our considered opinion that, apart from patient factors, applied surgical techniques and adequate speech training are the main factors affecting speech quality rather than the type of device used in tracheo-oesophageal fistula speech production.

Conclusions

The results lead to the following conclusions:

- Button-assisted oesophageal speech is louder and more readily intelligible in a noisy environment than injection-oesophageal speech. A few patients using button-assisted oesophageal speech are able to compete with normal laryngeal speakers so far as speech intelligibility is concerned.
- The SPC test is an objective and reliable method of estimating vocal communication ability, especially when combined with vocal intensity measurements.
- The SPC test, however, seems to be of far greater importance in determining patient speech quality than the measurement of maximum vocal intensity.
- Preliminary LTAS analysis results of running speech suggest a correlation between SPC and the spectral slope.

References

Gates GA et al. (1982) Current status of laryngectomee rehabilitation. I Results of therapy. Am J Otolaryngology 3:1–7

Schaeffer SD, Johns DF (1982) Attaining functional esophageal speech. Arch Otolaryngol 108:647–649

Schutte HK et al. (1985) Evaluation of speech with and without a "Groningen type" voice button. In: Speech Restoration via Voice Prosthesis. Int. Workshop, June 1984, Würzburg

The Postlaryngectomy Telephone Intelligibility Test (PLTT)

H. P. Zenner [1]

Assessments of different modes of alaryngeal speech require quantitative measurements of the relative intelligibility of individual speakers. Thus, the purpose of our investigation (Zenner 1984; Zenner and Pfrang 1986) was to establish an easy and rapid test system allowing the quantitative analysis and evaluation of voice restoration. Past investigations of the comparative intelligibility of alaryngeal speakers have assessed relative intelligibility by discriminatory procedures based on freely spoken single words (Hyman 1955; Shames et al. 1963; McChoskey and Mulligan 1963; Kalb and Carpenter 1981). We sought to assess the absolute intelligibility of alaryngeal speech modes with a discrimination test which would meet the required criteria for normal communicative tasks.

There are a number of audiological approaches to determine speech intelligibility. According to Carhart (1965), the patient's linguistic background is the most important selection criterion for any particular discrimination test. Linguistic background is a variable which is beyond the examiner's control in an open-response discrimination test (Carhart 1965). Thus, a closed response set has a decided advantage over an open one because all subjects, regardless of language background, must choose their responses from the same linguistic pool (Clark and Stemple 1982). Our discriminatory test system focuses on speech intelligibility as the most important parameter of voice restoration. Therefore, we investigated closed response sets compiled from phonetically-balanced linguistic pools: the Freiburg word list and the Marburg sentence list. Both lists are widely used in German-speaking countries for speech audiogramm purposes.

Initially, the laryngectomee says words and sentences directly (freely spoken) to an investigator with normal hearing but without visual contact. The listener writes down what he has understood, thus allowing quantitative calculations of the patient's intelligibility percentage. To investigate the validity of this approach, 63 laryngectomized speakers were judged by a panel of 20 investigators. Each patient was judged 8–12 times by 8–12 individual listeners. We were able to show (Zenner 1984; Zenner and Pfrang 1986) that the test results were reproducible in a statistically significant manner and that they were also independent of individual investigators. Both these factors are basic prerequisites for such a test system. On the other hand, bisyllables and direct listening did not enable a sufficient discrimination and ranking of the patient's relative intelligibility. Figure 1 shows that most speakers are correctly understood at a rate of 90%–100% when using

[1] Universitätsklinik und Poliklinik für Hals-, Nasen- und Ohrenkranke im Kopfklinikum, D-8700 Würzburg.

Speech Restoration Via Voice Prostheses
Edited by I. F. Herrmann

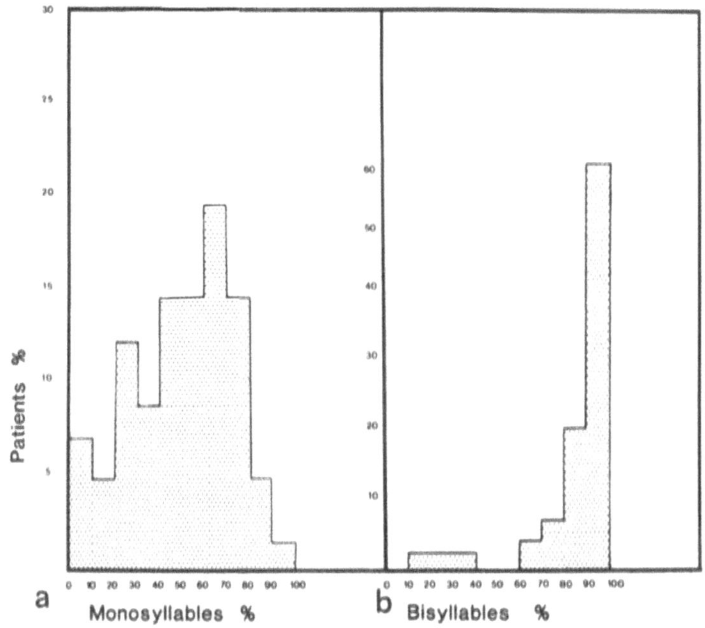

Fig. 1 a, b. Relative intelligibility of monosyllables and bisyllables. 63 laryngectomised speakers (oesophageal and TE-shunt speakers) were judged by 20 investigators with normal hearing. Each patient was judged 8–12 times by 8–12 investigators. Over 600 test situations with freely-spoken bisyllables (and numbers) gave an overall voice restoration with a 90–100% intelligibility rate. **b** Freely-spoken bisyllables and numbers clearly produce incorrectly positive intelligibility results. By contrast, monosyllables on a telephone produce mean percentage intelligibility scores that can differentiate individual speakers

bisyllables. This is identical to the rate of healthy individuals. Thus, freely-spoken bisyllables (and numbers) give positive intelligibility results which are incorrect!

To overcome these problems in relation to the audiological tests of Martin and Mussel (1979), words and sentences were attended by a continuous noise signal with a +6 dB competition-to-noise ratio (Jerger et al. 1968). We can show that the use of a competing noise background does provide a valid simulation of

Table 1. Examples of (**a**) random monosyllables and 5 random sentences used in a PLTT on a telephone, and (**b**) the linguistic pool providing patterns of similar words which eliminate preconceptions on the listener's behalf (statistically shown in the reliability values of 0.90–0.93)

a	Ring	Raum	**b**	Hund	Erz
	Schnee	Hang		Mund	Herz
	Spott	Hemd		Schlund	März
	Feld	Geist		Bund	Terz
	Farm	Kamm		Sund	Scherz

Geld allein macht nicht glücklich
Böse Menschen verdienen ihre Strafe
Mittwoch kommt uns Besuch passend
Ich bin nicht naß geworden
Uns're Eltern tanzen Wiener Walzer

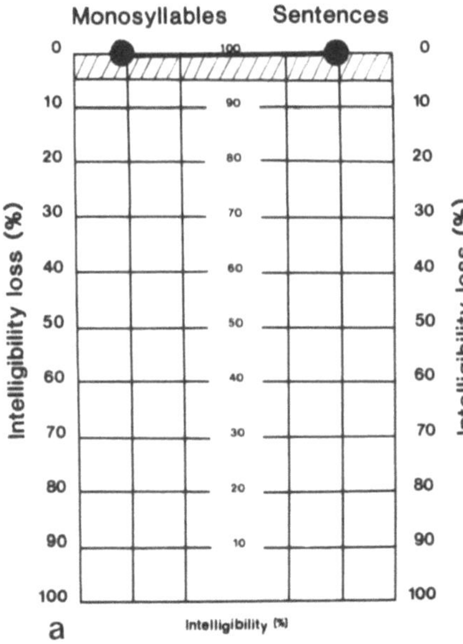

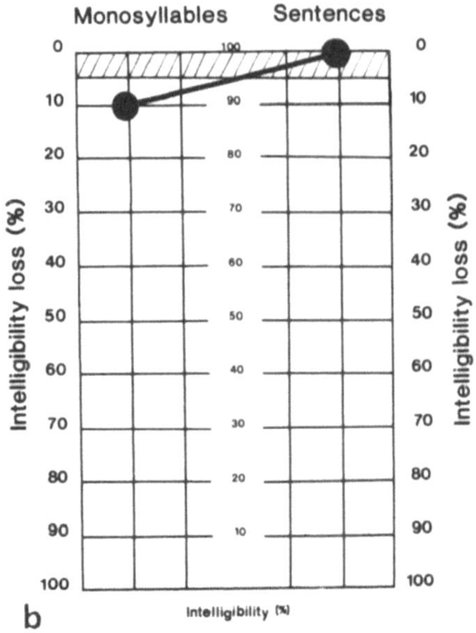

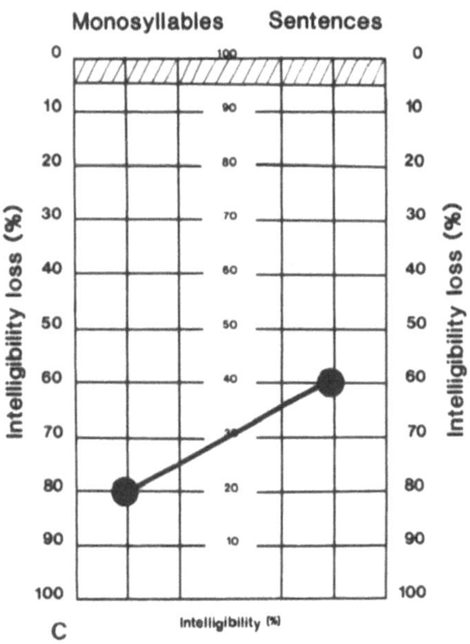

Fig. 2 a–c. Clinical application of the PLTT. The graph shows the intelligibility and intelligibility loss for monosyllables (*left*) and sentences (*right*). **a** Healthy speakers; no intelligibility loss, **b** typical laryngectomized speaker with primary TE-shunt, voice prosthesis, and myotomy (PLTT represents 80% of patients in this group): intelligibility loss is 0%–10%, and **c** typical laryngectomized speaker after 3 months of oesophageal speech training (PLTT represents 60% of patients in this group): intelligibility loss is 60%–80%. Note that PLTT is used similarly to a speech audiogram

real-life listening conditions. Furthermore, control measurements have revealed that these conditions are also created by using a telephone (Zenner 1984; Zenner and Pfrang 1986). Figure 1 demonstrates for example that, in contrast to freely spoken bisyllables and numbers, monosyllables on a telephone provide mean percentage intelligibility scores capable of differentiating individual speakers.

To investigate these questions more fully, we began to evaluate the extent to which individual Freiburg words and Marburg sentences are satisfactory predic-

Table 2. Principle of the PLTT (Post Laryngectomy Telephone Test) according to Zenner (1984)

Patient reads		Investigator hears
monosyllables and sentences	Telephone ⟶	% understanding?

tors of conversational speech intelligibility under telephone message-to-competition conditions. On the telephone, the reliability of monosyllables and sentences was 0.93 or 0.90, and 0.91 or 0.90 according to Spearman and Cronbach, respectively. The maximum value in these statistical tests was 1.0. Our values therefore show the high reliability of the word and sentence list used in our postlaryngectomy telephone intelligibility test. Furthermore, the 0.52 and 0.7 part per whole (p-w) discrimination values show that one monosyllable alone is 25% and one single sentence is 49% capable of predicting the correct rank of vocal rehabilitation. Psychological controls revealed that the PLT-test really does reproduce real-life listening situations (Zenner 1984; Zenner and Pfrang 1986). The test was therefore based on 20 monosyllables and 5 sentences (Table 1a). Furthermore, direct listening (a zero dB message-to-competition ratio) was not allowed and a noise background was obligatory. This condition is reproduced when using a telephone.

Thus, the postlaryngectomy telephone intelligibility test enables the exact prediction, assessment, and evaluation of speech intelligibility after laryngectomy. The test uses 20 changing monosyllables and 5 changing sentences under telephone conditions. Bisyllables, number, or freely spoken words must not be used as they give false results. The test is easily and rapidly performed. It is reproducible and independent of an investigator with normal hearing. Apart from a telephone and a word and sentence pool list (available on request; English version in preparation), no special equipment is required.

The laryngectomee slowly reads 20 random words and 5 random sentences on a telephone (Table 1a gives an example). The investigator writes down what he has understood. We can show that randomization and the use of similar word patterns (Table 1b) exclude any preconceptions the listener may have. A simple comparison between what the patient said and what the listener wrote enables the calculation of the speech intelligibility percentage and intelligibility loss. Figure 2 gives some typical examples of PLT-tests on oesophageal speakers and laryngectomees with a voice prosthesis. The results are given in graphical form as intelligibility loss. This allows a rapid evaluation of the patient's voice restoration.

In a test on 160 patients (Table 3), 10% of the oesophageal speakers had an intelligibility loss of less than 10% and could therefore use a telephone. This compares with 60% after a voice prosthesis has been inserted into a TE-shunt. A pri-

Table 3. Statistically controlled advantages of the PLTT according to Zenner (1984)

a) Exact measurement of conversational speech intelligibility (loss)
b) Easy and quick
c) Reproducible
d) Independent of investigator with normal hearing

Table 4. PLTT of 160 laryngectomees using different alaryngeal speech modes. The table indicates the number of patients (in %) with an intelligibility loss of less than 10% in the PLTT

	Esophageal speech	Secondary TP-shunt	Primary TP-shunt	
			−Myotomy	+Myotomy
Intelligibility loss <10%	10% (N=30)	60% (N=53)	61% (N=54)	82% (N=23)

mary technique including TE-shunt, voice prosthesis, and functional surgery of the hypopharynx allows more than 80% of patients to be understood on the telephone (Table 4).

References

Carhart R (1965) Problems in the measurement of speech discrimination. Arch Otolaryng 82:253–260

Clark JG, Stemple JC (1982) Assessment of three modes of alaryngeal speech with a synthetic sentence identification (SSI) task in varying message-to-competition ratios. J Speech Hearing Research 25:333

Hyman H (1955) An experimental study of artificial larynx and oesophageal speech. J Speech Hearing Disorders 20:291–299

Jerger J et al. (1968) A new approach to speech audiometry. J Speech Hearing Disorders 33:318–328

Kalb MB, Carpenter MA (1981) Individual speaker influence on relative intelligibility of oesophageal speech and artificial larynx speech. J Speech Hearing Disorders 46:77–80

Martin F, Mussell S (1979) The influence of pauses in the competing signal on synthetic sentence identification scores. J Speech Hearing Disorders 44:282–292

McChoskey RL, Mulligan M (1963) The relative intelligibility of oesophageal speech and artificial larynx speech. J Speech Hearing Disorders 28:37–41

Shames GH et al. (1963) Factors related to speech proficiency of the laryngectomized. J Speech Hearing Disorders 28:273–287

Zenner HP (1984) Ein Sprachverständlichkeitstest für Laryngektomierte. Paper presented at the annual convention of the Dt Ges Phon Pädaudiol, Reichenhall

Zenner HP, Pfrang H (1986) Ein einfacher Sprachverständlichkeitstest zur Beurteilung der Stimmrehabilitation des Laryngektomierten. Laryng Rhinol Otol 65:271–276

4 Years Experience of Voice Production and Deglutition Using Valve Prostheses

H. P. ZENNER [1] and I. F. HERRMANN [1]

Introduction

130 of our patients have undergone prosthetic voice restoration using primary or secondary tracheo-pharyngeal (TP) shunt techniques (Herrmann and Kley 1981; Zenner and Herrmann 1983; Herrmann et al. 1984). An objective analysis of the outcome of the procedure was made according to two major criteria: (1) the ability to swallow without aspiration, and (2) the production of vocal sounds enabling speech rehabilitation with less than 10% intelligibility loss in the PLT-test according to Zenner (1984; this volume, p. 148). Furthermore, the effect of radiotherapy was evaluated on each of these two criteria.

The Secondary TP-Puncture

In 53 patients, we performed an outpatient endoscopic procedure using a large oesophagoscope (this volume, p. 43). A puncture needle (Koss Company, Geisenheim, W. Germany) is introduced by the surgeon through the posterior tracheal wall into the distal end of the rotated endoscope. After removal, the puncture needle is replaced by a silicon stent. The stent is held back by an inner retention collar. After 2 weeks, a suitable voice prosthesis is inserted into the puncture site. Speech intelligibility and intelligibility loss were determined according to Zenner (1984; this volume, p. 148) using the PLT-test (PLTT). 60% of the patients developed speech with an intelligibility loss of less than 10%, whereas only 10% of the controls, i.e., the oesophageal speakers belonged to this group. In the PLTT, healthy students had an intelligibility loss of less than 5%, which represents the normal degree of variation (Table 1). From this it was concluded that the secondary TP-shunt technique enables a considerable improvement on oesophageal speech.

Despite this, the results also represent a considerable failure. Therefore, intratracheal and intrapharyngeal air pressure flow and resistance were determined during postoperative visits. Furthermore, pharyngeal mechanics were visualized during speech production by transfistular contrast radiography. Voice failures produced severe intrapharyngeal pressure and reduced mucosal motility which in

[1] Universitätsklinik und Poliklinik für Hals-, Nasen- und Ohrenkranke im Kopfklinikum, D-8700 Würzburg.

Speech Restoration Via Voice Prostheses
Edited by I. F. Herrmann

Table 1. Intelligibility loss in 160 patients with different alaryngeal speech modes. Intelligibility loss (IL) was determined using the PLT-Test (Post-Laryngectomy Telephone Test) according to Zenner (1984; this volume, p. 148). The table indicates the percentage of patients with an IL of less than 10%

	Oesophageal speech	Secondary TP-shunt	Primary TP-shunt	
			−myotomy	+myotomy
Intelligibility loss <10%	10% (N=30)	60% (N=53)	61% (N=54)	82% (N=23)

turn created excessive air flow resistance. Due to pharyngeal resistance, transprosthetic air flow is inhibited by the hypopharynx and voice production is either weakened or totally inhibited (Herrmann et al. 1984).

22 laryngectomees were punctured after a full course of postoperative radiation therapy. 10 of these patients had aspiration problems resulting from insufficiencies or pharyngeal edemas. No aspiration was found in 31 patients who had not undergone radiation therapy. It is therefore concluded that the secondary shunt technique (in contrast to the primary technique) cannot be recommended for patients who have undergone radiation therapy.

Glottoplasty – The Primary Technique

To overcome these problems, we developed a procedure which (1) decreases airflow resistance, (2) creates a voice shunt during wide field laryngectomy, (3) uses a low pressure valve prosthesis (Koss Company, Geisenheim, W. Germany), and (4) creates a reproducibly uniform tracheostoma (Herrmann and Kley 1981; Zenner and Herrmann 1983; Herrmann et al. 1984).

During complete transection of the trachea, a dorsal mucosal flap is prepared bevelling the tracheal cut. A defined perforation is incised into the skin-fascia flap allowing the trachea and the dorsal mucosal flap to be sutured on to the skin. This procedure creates a uniform tracheostoma matching the size of the patient's finger.

The creation of a tracheo-hypopharyngeal shunt in conjunction with wide field laryngectomy is a quick and easy procedure. The pharyngeal and the posterior tracheal walls are simply perforated with a puncture needle so that the stenting silicon tube can be drawn into the newly formed shunt.

Anatomical stenoses must be avoided to reduce intrapharyngeal airflow resistance. In addition, a lateral myotomy of the circular muscle fibres near Killian's inlet is performed. To avoid the dorsal hypopharyngeal muscle bulk (see p. 43 in this volume), the outer pharyngeal muscle layer is incised dorso-medially. Landmarks not to be compromised by this type of outer myotomy are the superior nerves as well as the intramural blood vessels (Herrmann et al. 1984).

Two weeks after laryngectomy, a low pressure valve prosthesis (ESKA-Herrmann) is inserted into the shunt.

Table 2. Transfistular aspiration of 130 patients with TP-shunt and voice prosthesis. Note how major problems only occur if the shunt is created *after* radiation therapy (cf. text). If the shunt is formed *prior* to radiation therapy (i.e., using the primary technique), the consolidated TP-fistula is not usually affected by later radiation. A low aspiration rate of less than 3% results

Radiation	Secondary TP-shunt	Primary TP-shunt
None	0/31	0/35
Before shunt creation	10/22	–
After shunt creation	–	2/42

77 patients underwent the primary shunt procedure: (1) 54 individuals without and, (2) 23 individuals with a dorsal myotomy. In the series of 54 patients who did not undergo a myotomy, 33 laryngectomies (61%) achieved fluent speech with the PLTT (Zenner 1984; this volume, p. 148) with an intelligibility loss of less than 10%. This result is similar to that obtained by the secondary technique (60%) and better than that obtained by oesophageal speech (10%). In contrast to this, the series of 23 patients who underwent additional intraoperative dorsal myotomy included 19 patients (82%) who attained excellent speech with an intelligibility loss of less than 10%. Therefore 10% of oesophageal speakers, 60% of prosthetic speakers without myotomy, and 80% of patients with voice prostheses and pharyngeal myotomy mastered the telephone with a 90%–100% intelligibility level.

In contrast to the secondary shunt technique, postoperative radiation therapy did not induce serious aspiration problems out of 77 patients. The reason for this is that radiation of the consolidated shunt (i.e., the primary technique) does not disrupt the sealing function of the shunt whereas the formation of a fistula in radiated tissue (i.e., the secondary technique) can lead to considerable leakage (Table 2).

Leakage, aspiration, or speech loss due to prosthesis damage occurs for most patients every 3–15 months. A simple prosthesis removal easily overcomes this normal problem.

The low failure rate and relative freedom from complications found in patients who have undergone primary voice rehabilitation and pharyngeal myotomy have been observed now for a period of over two years. This was for patients with excessive primary resections, radiation therapy, and varying socio-economic status.

Finally, the primary shunt technique can be combined successfully with pharynx reconstructions by employing myocutaneous island flaps or gastric transpositions.

References

Herrmann IF, Kley W (1981) The glottoplasty. In: Surjan L (ed) Proc. World Congr. ORL, Budapest

Herrmann IF, Zenner HP (1984) Erfahrungen mit der Blom-Singer-Prothese. HNO 32:286–293

Herrmann IF, Buchwald J, Zenner HP (1984) Die Glottoplastik. HNO 32:294–301

Zenner HP (1984) Ein Sprachverständlichkeitstest für Laryngektomierte. Paper presented at the annual meeting of the Dt Ges Phon Pädaudiol, Reichenhall

Zenner HP, Herrmann IF (1983) A new versatile technique for primary and secondary surgical voice restoration following laryngectomy. In: Ward P, Berman W (eds) Proc Acad Plast Reconstr Surg, Los Angeles Mosby. St. Louis, pp 1102–1106

Chapter 6 Speech Training, Intelligibility and Psychosocial Aspects

Speech Training of Oesophageal Voice with a Button

E. F. M. BORS, G. H. A. DE BOER and H. K. SCHUTTE [1]

Introduction

As a rule, 2 kinds of oesophageal voice are trained in the Groningen ENT clinic after laryngectomy:

1. Oesophageal voice with the injection method (Moolenaar-Bijl 1953)
2. Oesophageal voice with the button (Nijdam et al. 1982).

ad 1. For the injection method, air is compressed in the mouth and pharynx by tongue and jaw movements. This is achieved mainly by sounding of the occlusive consonants, p, t, and k. During occlusion, the pressure in the mouth and pharynx will be high enough to allow a certain amount of air to be injected into the oesophagus. In this way, a small air reservoir can be created under the cricopharyngeal muscle. In this region the so-called pseudoglottis is located. The patient can make the oesophageal pressure rise so high that a small amount of air can escape into the pharyngeal cavity, causing the pseudoglottis to vibrate. This is how the oesophageal voice source is vibrated. The outgoing sound is formed by the shape of the vocal tract and articulators.

ad 2. For the button, air is supplied from the lungs and not through the mouth. In this case, the patient must close his tracheostoma with the thumb or fingers. The air flows from the lungs through the trachea and the tracheo-oesophageal shunt into the oesophagus. The pressure in the oesophagus reservoir is also supplied by the lungs so that air can escape through the pseudoglottis, causing the vibrations known as oesophageal voice. Whether using injection oesophageal voice or button-oesophageal voice, the sound source for both is located at the pharyngo-oesophageal segment. The only difference is in the method of air supply. As the amount of air supplied by the injection method is restricted, the maximum duration of the phonation is consequently rather short. By contrast the air reservoir in the oesophagus with button-oesophageal voice can be constantly refilled through the button. Because of the large air reservoir formed by the lungs, maximum phonation duration is longer than with the injection method. Breath control also differs in both methods due to the different sources of air supply. For the injection method, the patient must learn to exspire through the tracheostoma as quietly as possible. Conversely, when using a button, the patient must learn to allow the air stream through the button in a normal relaxed way. As the speech training of injection-oesophageal voice is already well-known, the speech therapy of button-oesophageal voice is discussed in this paper.

[1] Academic Hospital Groningen, 9700 RB Groningen, The Netherlands.

Speech Restoration Via Voice Prostheses
Edited by I. F. Herrmann

Table 1. Steps in the speech training of button-oesophageal voices

1.	Good posture
2.	Relaxing exercises for head and neck
3.	Normal inhalation
4.	Closing of the tracheostoma
5.	Phonation
6.	Words beginning with a vowel; sentences; series
7.	Refinement of speech

The speech training procedure is as follows (Table 1):

1. Firstly, we emphasize good body and head posture.
2. Secondly, the patient does specific exercises to relax the head and neck region.
3. Thirdly, the patient is instructed to inhale in a normal relaxed way, i.e., not too deeply.
4. Fourthly, the patient is taught to close his tracheostoma with the thumb or with 1 or 2 fingers. A gauze or a foam band can be used for this purpose. Most patients find it difficult to occlude the stoma in the correct place. If the stoma is only partly completed, a hissing sound is heard during phonation impeding voice intelligibility. In order to be sure as to whether the patient can phonate with a properly occluded stoma in the first place, the speech trainer may occlude the patient's stoma.
5. In the fifth step, the patient can start to phonate by simply exhaling once the stoma is closed. The easiest way to do this is by producing an open vowel, if this can be produced easily. It sounds similar to a low relaxed oesophageal voice. In order to avoid a plopping sound at the end of phonation, the expiratory movement must stop before the stoma is opened. If necessary, the patient is instructed to breathe with low abdominal respiration.
6. The sixth step is to teach the patient to speak words beginning with an initial vowel once he has proved that he can easily produce an open vowel. As soon as these can be produced in a relaxed way, sentences and series are trained. The utterances can grow longer and longer. The patient's attention is directed towards the production of a relaxed sound and good breath management.
7. The final step, depending on the patient's technical skills, is to pay increasing attention to intonation and loudness. We use interrogative and exclamatory sentences and we also read texts.

We will now briefly discuss the advantages and disadvantages of button-oesophageal speech compared with injection-oesophageal voice. One advantage is that the patient can speak more fluently. Phonation lasts longer and more syllables can be produced without interruption. Moreover, the patient has a greater variation of intonation and volume. The voice is louder, easier to learn, and more rapidly available. Finally, the voice is made on the basis of normal expiration as with laryngeal speech. The disadvantages are that the patients always need to use one hand to occlude the stoma and the button needs to be regularly replaced.

Finally, we would like to present some results from our follow-up study (Table 2): We have found that if a patient can use button-oesophageal voice, he

Table 2. Success rate of useful oesophageal voice after 1 week and after 6 months

	Patients without button (N=49)	Patients with button (N=22)	
	Injection voice	Injection voice	Button voice
1 week	47%	41%	73%
6 months	82%	73%	95%

will often speak usefully shortly after the operation. In our patient group 73% had a usable voice within this period of time. If a patient only learns the injection method, 47% attain a usable voice. 41% of the button-oesophageal speakers attain a usable voice with the injection method. We wish to draw your attention to the fact that useful button-oesophageal voice is of a better quality than useful injection-oesophageal voice. After 6 months, both voices are used in an acceptable way by most patients: 95% of the button-oesophageal speakers attained an acceptable button-oesophageal voice; after the same period, 73% of these speakers also attained an acceptable injection-oesophageal voice. In patients using the injection method without a button this was 82%. When patients acquire more skill in using injection-oesophageal voice during the postoperative year, they often prefer this kind of speech to button-oesophageal speech because they are able to keep both hands free while speaking. Furthermore, the regular replacement of the button is increasingly felt to be a disadvantage.

Conclusions

From the results of our follow-up study, we may conclude that button-oesophageal voice is of great value for the initial training of substitute voice. After several months when acceptable injection-oesophageal voice has been acquired, however, patients often prefer to use this kind of voice. This is the reason why we train both button-oesophageal and injection-oesophageal voice.

References

Nijdam HF et al. (1982) A new prosthesis for voice rehabilitation after laryngectomy. Arch Otorhinolaryngol 237:27–33

Moolenaar-Bijl AJ (1953) The importance of certain consonants in esophageal voice after laryngectomy. Ann Otol Rhinol Laryngol 62:979–989

Intelligibility and Psycho-Social Adjustment. A Comparison Between Patients with Oesophageal Voice and Patients with a Voice Prosthesis

H. Pfrang [1], H. de Maddalena [2], R. Schohe [2], J. Blaha [2], R. Piroth [1] and H. P. Zenner [2]

In this study, the results of 2 voice restoration methods are compared: oesophageal speech and surgical voice restoration via voice prosthesis (Herrmann prosthesis). Three criteria were employed to evaluate the results: (a) intelligibility, (b) the patients' own rating of how well different target persons understood him, and (c) general psycho-social adjustment. The working hypothesis that "patients with a prosthesis have better results than oesophageal speakers in all respects" is examined. Test intelligibility is assessed by using the post-laryngectomy telephone test (PLTT, Zenner, this volume, p. 148). The results are shown in Table 1.

Average intelligibility of prosthesis patients ranges from 63%–70% for monosyllables and from 83%–86% for sentences. Average intelligibility of oesophageal speakers ranges from 31%–53% for monosyllables and from 59%–70% for sentences. In all but one aspect, the "prosthesis" group achieved significantly higher scores on the different scales of intelligibility and in a variety of different situations. There is no difference for prosthesis patients between visual and nonvisual contact situations. By contrast, oesophageal speakers become more intelligible when listeners can see them.

The PLTT is an objective measurement of speech intelligibility for clinical purposes. In normal daily life, however, a communication partner can get used to the patient's speech. Therefore, an assessment was made as to how intelligible the patient thought he was to various different target persons. He was asked: "How well do you think your speech is understood by the following persons?" The patient had to rate how well he thought he was understood on a 5 point scale ranging from "very poorly" to "very well". The percentage of patients who rated their intelligibility as "very well" or "rather well" is shown in Table 2.

Within their own immediate family (spouse, children) the majority considered that they were well understood. There were no significant differences between the "oesophageal" and "prosthesis" groups and no common trend emerged. Outside the family circle there is a dramatic decrease in perceived intelligibility among oesophageal speakers compared with prosthesis patients. In general, the "prosthesis" group has a higher percentage of intelligibility and the differences are significant in 3 cases. Only about one quarter of the oesophageal speakers (23%–31%) believe that their best friend, an acquaintance, a neighbor or a clerk understands them well. This compares with about half the prosthesis patients (41%–63%). For the majority of oesophageal speakers, satisfactory intelligibility is re-

[1] Psychologisches Institut der Universität, D-8700 Würzburg.
[2] Universitätsklinik und Poliklinik für Hals-, Nasen- und Ohrenkranke im Kopfklinikum, D-8700 Würzburg.

Speech Restoration Via Voice Prostheses
Edited by I. F. Herrmann

Table 1. Test intelligibility of "oesophageal voice" compared to "voice prosthesis"

Test Situation Listener	Average percent understood		
	Oesophageal N=15	Prosthesis N=46	Significance
1. Test: 20 monosyllables			
1.1. Situation: with visual contact			
Listener	53%	69%	*
Family member	50%	70%	*
1.2. Situation: without visual contact			
Listener	40%	70%	***
Family member	41%	68%	**
Listener on telephone	31%	54%	**
2. Test: 25 monosyllables with difficult sounds			
Situation: without visual contact			
Listener	40%	69%	***
Family member	31%	63%	**
Listener on telephone	40%	56%	*
3. Test: 5 sentences			
Situation: without visual contact			
Listener	59%	85%	**
Family member	70%	83%	ns
Listener on telephone	65%	86%	*

Note 1: Method: Patient reads words or sentences, listeners write down, what they have understood

Note 2: Coding: Each correctly understood word gains 1 point, partially understood sentences also 1 point, and whole sentences 2 points

Note 3: Significance of difference: t-test, one-tailed; ns = not significant; * = $p < 0.05$; ** = $p < 0.01$; *** = $p < 0.001$

Table 2. Patient's perceived intelligibility according to target person for "oesophageal voice" and "voice prosthesis"

Target person	Percentage of patients rating intelligibility "very well" or "rather well"		
	Oesophageal	Prosthesis	Significance
Spouse	75%	85%	ns
Children	92%	68%	ns
Physician	47%	72%	*
Best friend	31%	63%	*
Acquaintance	23%	53%	*
Neighbor	31%	49%	ns
Clerk	25%	41%	ns
Partner on telephone	36%	56%	ns

Note: t-test, one-tailed; ns = not significant; * = $p < 0.05$; sample sizes vary according to target person

Table 3. A comparison between patients with oesophageal voice and patients with a voice prosthesis in terms of psycho-social adjustment

Scale	Mean and standard deviation		
	Oesophageal N=19	Prosthesis N=50	Significance
Social activities	21.3 10.4	23.3 9.8	ns
Life satisfaction	17.5 2.5	17.8 3.1	ns
Loneliness	15.2 4.0	13.5 3.3	*
Perceived decrease in quality of life	22.8 5.6	21.5 6.3	ns

Note: t-test, one-tailed; ns = not significant, * <0.05; a higher mean indicates more average agreement

stricted to the family. This is not true for the majority of prosthesis patients. We examined whether this also influenced psycho-social adjustment. The results are shown in Table 3.

See Pfrang (this volume, p. 165) for a more detailed description of the scales. There are no significant differences between the 2 groups regarding "social activities", "satisfaction in life", and "perceived decrease in quality of life". Oesophageal speakers achieve a significantly higher mean on the "loneliness" scale, which indicates a greater sense of social isolation. In general, however, the increased intelligibility derived from prosthesis voice restoration does not greatly influence psycho-social adjustment. These are only preliminary results pending further research.

Social and Psychosocial Aspects of Vocal Rehabilitation in Laryngectomized Patients – Preliminary Results

H. PFRANG [1]

Clinical observation indicates that voice acceptance depends on the method of restoration and that the personality and interpersonal relations of the laryngectomee might well affect the success of rehabilitation programmes. A review of the literature reveals a dearth of empirical and controlled research in this area. The Department of Otolaryngology and the Department of Psychology at Wuerzburg University are currently trying to determine the psycho-social aspects of different methods of voice restoration and general social adjustment. We have tried to answer two questions: (1) What socio-psychological factors influence voice restoration via prosthesis compared with other methods of voice restoration? (2) How relevant is intelligibility as a factor in patient communication and social adaptability?

1. Correlation of Different Voice Restoration Methods

The most important advantage of prosthesis voice restoration over oesophageal speech is the significantly increased intelligibility (Pfrang et al., this volume, p. 162). For example, average test intelligibility without visual contact increases from 40%–69% for 25 words with difficult sounds. This difference is due to the fact that one third of the patients, who should have learned oesophageal speech were not able to do so. Other investigators found a similar proportion of oesophageal speech failures (Salmon 1979); the most relevant single factor being lack of motivation (Shanks 1979). In this study, no significant correlation was found between intelligibility and motivation along prosthesis patients. However, high correlations were sometimes found among oesophageal speakers. If further research corroborates our work, one major advantage of prosthesis voice restoration would surely be that the achievement of good intelligibility does not depend on such psychological factors as motivation and learning.

Different voice restoration methods also tend to determine the extent to which the voice is accepted. No alaryngeal voice will attain the acceptance level of the laryngeal voice (Bennett and Weinberg 1973; Clark and Stemple 1982). Listeners consider pulmonary oesophageal voice via prosthesis to be more pleasant than artificial larynx and oesophageal voice (Clark and Stemple 1982). Acceptance levels in this study are not derived from universal criteria but from the attitudes and be-

[1] Psychologisches Institut der Universität, D-8700 Würzburg.

Speech Restoration Via Voice Prostheses
Edited by I. F. Herrmann

Table 1. Social reaction and emotional acceptance of voice impairment in terms of the different methods for voice restoration (means and standard deviations)

Variable	Control group No. of patients	Laryngectomized patients Method of voice restoration:			Significance of difference between "Prosthesis" and others		
		Artificial larynx	Oesophageal voice	Prosthesis	IV–I	IV–II	IV–III
	N=6 I	N=6 II	N=19 III	N=50 IV			
1. Social reaction							
Tracheostoma, conspicuousness	–	8.6	7.2	7.6	–	ns	ns
	–	2.3	2.4	2.4			
Voice, conspicuousness and rejection	6.7	12.4	8.7	8.2	ns	**	ns
	0.6	5.0	3.1	2.8			
Others often ask me to repeat myself	1.8	2.8	2.7	2.1	ns	**	***
	1.0	0.4	0.5	0.7			
Others have to listen very carefully to understand me	1.7	2.7	2.8	2.3	ns	ns	*
	0.8	0.5	0.4	0.7			
2. Coping							
Voice rejection	5.3	7.4	7.3	6.6	ns	ns	ns
	1.5	2.3	2.1	2.0			
Talks only, if he is forced to	1.7	2.5	1.8	1.7	ns	*	ns
	0.8	0.8	0.9	0.8			
Talks considerably less than before	1.5	3.0	2.4	2.4	**	ns	ns
	0.8	0.0	0.8	0.8			
Talks only about important things	1.2	2.3	2.2	1.9	*	ns	ns
	0.4	1.0	0.7	0.7			

N.B.: A high score indicates agreement, and a low score disagreement; statistical test; t-test, two-tailed; ns = not significant, * = $p<0.05$, ** = $p<0.01$, *** = $p<0.001$

havior patterns of the patient and other persons. The results are given in Table 1.

One working hypothesis was that prosthesis patients have a higher „social conspicuousness and rejection because of the stoma“ than oesophageal speakers. Closing the stoma with a finger would probably attract attention to the patient's stoma, possibly increasing both conspicuousness and rejection at the same time. Oesophageal speakers proved to have the lowest mean, however, and there was no significant difference between the groups. Finger occlusion of the stoma did not entail a greater degree of conspicuousness, more staring, etc.

To determine the degree of handicap experienced after laryngectomy via different methods of voice restoration, a comparison was made with cancer patients who had not undergone total laryngectomy. As could be expected, this „control group“ had the lowest scores for all speech variables. Artificial larynx speakers experienced more social conspicuousness and rejection. They also rejected their own voices more than patients in the „control group“. These differences were not significant as the test samples were small. However, artificial larynx patients are asked to repeat themselves significantly ($p<0.5$) more often and others are obliged to listen more attentively. They therefore talk considerably less and only speak about essential things. These differences are also significant ($p<0.1$) for oesophageal speakers. Despite the greater sample size, the „prosthesis“ group differs in only two variables from the „control group“: Prosthesis patients talk considerably less than before and talk only about essential things. In comparison with the „control group“, the degree of impairment, handicap and nonacceptance seems somewhat less for prosthesis patients.

A comparison between the groups of alaryngeal speakers shows significantly better results in some variables for prosthesis patients. Pulmonary oesophageal speakers are less socially conspicuous and face less rejection than artificial larynx speakers. They are less frequently asked to repeat themselves and find that they ave to reduce their speech to essentials less often. There are two significant differences between the „oesophageal voice“ and „prosthesis“ groups: Other people ask oesophageal speakers to repeat themselves more often and have to listen more carefully.

From a psychological point of view, voice restoration via prosthesis seems more favorable for two reasons: good motivation and learning capacity are less important than with oesophageal voice, and intelligibility and acceptance will be higher. Psycho-social adjustment factors are especially relevant to the planning of rehabilitation programmes.

2. Psycho-Social Adjustment Correlations Among Prosthesis Patients

The correlations between four psycho-social adjustment factors and other selected variables in prosthesis patients are shown in Table 2. The level of adjustment is indicated by the „frequency of social activities“ (14 items; e.g., small talk with neighbors, visiting friends, going to meetings, going to bars, going out on errands), „Life satisfaction“ (12 items; e.g., patient agrees that the future will be happier; disagrees with the statement that: „Sometimes I don't care whether I live or die“, „loneliness“ (10 items; e.g., feeling isolated, no one to talk to), and „perceived decrease in life quality after laryngectomy“ (17 items; whereby a high score indicates that one's self-esteem and enjoyment of various areas of life and social integration had „got worse“).

There is no significant correlation between „test intelligibility“ and adjustment, and there was only one significant correlation with perceived intelligibility (target person: an acquaintance). Patients, who experience greater intelligibility, report more social activities. In general, intelligibility only slightly affects the social adjustment of prosthesis patients. One major social factor is the reaction experienced towards the tracheostoma and voice impairment. „Conspicuousness and rejection because of stoma“ correlates significantly and negatively with „frequency of social activities“ and „life satisfaction“, and positively with „decrease in life quality“. „Conspicuousness and rejection because of voice“ correlates in a positively significant way with „loneliness“ and „decrease in life quality“. Patients, who feel both conspicuous and rejected, tend to engage in fewer social ac-

Table 2. Correlations between 4 aspects of psychosocial adjustment and intelligibility, social reaction, and coping among laryngectomized patients with voice prosthesis (N = 50; Sperman's rho)

Variable	Psychosocial adjustment			
	Frequency of social activities	Life satis-faction	Lone-liness	Perceived decrease in life quality after laryngectomy
Test intelligibility (25 words, no visual contact)	0.18 ns	0.00 ns	−0.08 ns	0.02 ns
Perceived intelligibility (acquaintance)	0.30[a]	0.05 ns	−0.10 ns	−0.12 ns
Tracheostoma and neck breathing, social conspicuousness, and rejection	−0.39[b]	−0.31[a]	0.23 ns	0.37[b]
Voice, social conspicuousness, and rejection	−0.19 ns	−0.26 ns	0.43[b]	0.31[a]
Voice rejection	−0.33[a]	−0.37[b]	0.25 ns	0.28[a]
Withdrawal from talking	−0.34[a]	−0.18 ns	0.22 ns	0.19 ns
Positive evaluation of laryngectomy	0.09 ns	0.43[b]	−0.48[b]	−0.17 ns
Alternatives to loss of employment	0.16 ns	0.31[a]	−0.20 ns	−0.15 ns

N.B. Two-tailed test of significance; ns = not significant
[a] $p<0.05$
[b] $p<0.01$

tivities and gain less satisfaction from life. They feel lonelier and more isolated and report a greater decrease in the quality of their lives after laryngectomy in a number of spheres.

Another major factor dealt with here is the capacity to cope with impairment. A patient's negative attitude towards his own voice („voice rejection“) reduces his active participation in social activities and his satisfaction with life. This in turn increases his sense of impairment in the quality of his life significantly.

„Withdrawal from talking“ (only about essential things, less than before, etc.) reduces social activities significantly. „Positive evaluation of laryngectomy“ (e.g., it's better to have a longer impaired life than to die earlier) correlates positively with „life satisfaction“ and negatively with „loneliness“. „Alternatives to loss of employment“ (e.g., hobbies, more time for family life) also correlates positively with „life satisfaction“.

The degree of psycho-social adjustment does not seem to depend on the mere facts of laryngectomy and voice impairment but on individual and social reactions. Further research will determine the aforementioned variables more precisely by using larger samples. Similarly, relations with other variables, such as social support, will also be studied in greater detail. A clinical psychologist may be useful in helping the selection and rehabilitation of laryngectomized patients. He can teach the patient how to cope with possible preoperative and postoperative emotional crises, long term voice impairment, loss of employment, etc. He can also counsel the patient's family. Another publication is currently being prepared concerning the criteria and techniques of psychological intervention.

References

Bennett S, Weinberg B (1973) Acceptability ratings of normal, oesophageal and artificial larynx speech. J Speech Hearing Research 16:608–614

Clark JG, Stemple JC (1982) Assessment of three modes of alaryngeal speech with a synthetic sentence identification (SSI) task in varying message-to-competition ratios. J Speech Hearing Research 25:333–338

Salmon SJ (1979) Factors that may interfere with acquiring esophageal speech. In: Keith RJ, Darley FC (eds) Laryngectomee rehabilitation. College Hill Press, Houston, pp 379–402

Shanks JC (1979) Essentials for alaryngeal speech-psychology and physiology. In: Keith RJ, Darley FC (eds) Laryngectomee rehabilitation. College Hill Press, Houston, pp 469–490

Chapter 7 Fingerless Voice Restoration

Experiences with Surgical Voice Restoration

R. M. Tiwari, H. D. Vuyk and G. B. Snow[1]

Patients and Methods

Roughly 150 total laryngectomies are performed throughout the Netherlands each year. In our Department of Otolaryngology at the Free University Hospital, an average of 20 total laryngectomies are performed a year. These are largely when radiation treatment has failed or for larger (T_3, T_4) tumors. Speech therapy and the oesophageal voice technique are well developed in the Netherlands. 60% of our laryngectomized patients have good oesophageal voice and can communicate satisfactorily. Another 30% have some form of voice and 10% fail to develop any voice at all. From 1979 to 1983 we therefore attempted to rehabilitate a total of 41 patients by the Staffieri technique (Tables 1 and 2). The method was attractive as it involves a one-stage technique and does not interfer with the oncological principles of primary tumor surgery. Besides, other methods can still be used where necessary. The procedure of the technique is well-known. We kept to Staffieri's recommendation and did not exceed the 5 mm length of the tracheo-oesophageal fistula.

Table 1. Material and methods

Total number of patients 41
Males 39, females 2
Average age 58.3 years (41 to 78 years)
Period of study 1979 through 1983
Size of "neoglottis" 4.5 to 5 mm

Table 2. Factors pertaining to the primary laryngeal lesion

Localization – glottic and/or supraglottic	
Pathology – Well to moderately differentiated squamous cell carcinomas	
(Supraglottic lesions were unsuitable for partial horizontal supraglottic laryngectomy)	
Recurrence after radiotherapy	– 21
En bloc radical neck dissection	– 17 – two bilateral
Postoperative radiotherapy	– 4
All excisions were radical	

[1] De Boelelaan 1117, 1007 Amsterdam, The Netherlands.

Speech Restoration Via Voice Prostheses
Edited by I. F. Herrmann

Table 3. Results of total laryngectomy using Staffieri's technique

Author		Number of patients	Revision	Percentage of success
Bailey	1982	50	21	50
Calearo	1981	63	14	68
Draf	1980	34	12	50
Gatti	1981	10	4	70
Hybasek	1982	28	8	65
Kuske	1981	19	4	65
McConnel	1982	13	7	50
Navaratil	1981	12	–	50
Sisson	1980	26	8	65
Staffieri	1979	105	36	91
Steiner	1980	50	–	43
Tiwari	1982	32	3	50

Results

A retrospective analysis of the results showed that 75% of the patients initially benefited from this procedure and could eat, drink, and talk. During the next 12 months, however, one third of these patients developed increased aspiration. The remaining 50% continued to lead a satisfactory normal life without any obvious complaints (Table 3). Revision surgery did not help to solve the aspiration problems. It also confirmed that the original operation had been carried out exactly as recommended and that the neoglottis had not changed structurally. We therefore discontinued revision surgery and solved the problem by placing a Groningen type button into the fistula with satisfactory results. The reason for the aspiration, however, later became apparent. A stenosis of the neoglottis only developed in 3 patients and all these 3 were able to lead a normal life again after endoscopic revision. In 4 patients, the neoglottis was closed and oesophageal speech restored after speech therapy.

Discussion

From this we learned that, as with any other surgical technique, a strict selection of cases is important. Proper preoperative preparation is likewise essential. Successful results were obtained even though half of our cases had been primarily radiated. However, the radiotherapy dosage is relevant. When large tumors are removed and limited pharyngeal mucosa and musculature remains one can expect problems. Accompanying neck dissection did not significantly affect the results. It was striking to note that when such complications as salivary fistula developed they took much longer to heal in a patient with a tracheo-oesophageal shunt (Staffieri neoglottis) than in one with a conventional laryngectomy. We consider this a major drawback of the technique (Table 4). Studies were conducted in our Department together with the Department of Gastro-Enterology on the mano-

Table 4. Salivary fistula after total laryngectomy

	Conventional broad-field laryngectomy	Laryngectomy according to Staffieri
Primary surgery	13%	36%
Surgery for recurrence after radiotherapy	20%	41%

metric pressure levels of these patients. The results suggest that the aspiration problems in some individuals may be related to incomplete relaxation in the pharynx above the neoglottis at the socalled upper oesophageal sphincter level. The results also suggest insufficient coordination of the musculature and cricopharyngeal sphincter leading to a stasis of the bolus above the neoglottis. Cricopharyngeal myotomy can certainly be recommended as a measure to accompany any future surgical procedure. Electroglottographic studies conducted by Lecluse tend to confirm the fluency of neoglottic speech and indeed patients prefer this to oesophageal voice. Endoscopic examination after surgery and xeroradiography has shown that pharyngeal musculature and mucosa adapt remarkably well to produce pseudo-vocal folds which then largely serve as the sound source.

Our experience with the prosthesis is limited as we only used it in those cases where oesophageal voice failed to develop and where the patient was generally fit enough to take care of his prosthesis. Although we have come a long way since the first attempts 11 decades ago, many problems still remain to be solved and many questions remain unanswered.

References

Bailay BJ (1982) Neoglottic reconstruction: The Staffieri technique. In: Sekey A (ed) Electroacoustic analysis and enhancement of alaryngeal speech. Thomas, Springfield, Ill

Calearo CV (1981) Total laryngectomy with tracheopharyngeal fistula (neoglottis). Ann Otol Rhinol Laryngol 90:217–221

Draf W (1980) Persönliche Mitteilungen. Therapeutische Umschau 37/12:1117–1127

Gatti WM (1981) Creation of the phonatory neoglottis. Preliminary experiences with ten cases. Acta Otolaryngol 91:305–312

Hybasek I (1982) Neoglottis phonatoria, our experiments. 10th congress of the Union of European Phoniatricians, Prague

Kuske I (1981) Erfahrungen mit der Methode von Staffieri zur Wiederherstellung der Stimme nach totaler Laryngektomie. Laryng Rhinol Otol 60:373–375

Lecluse FLE (1981) Electroglottographic studies of Staffieri neoglottis. The Laryngoscope 91:971–975

McConnel FMS (1982) Neoglottis reconstruction following total laryngectomy. The Emroy Experience. Otolaryngol Head Neck Surg 90:569–575

Navratil J (1981) Our experience with laryngectomy according to Staffieri (neoglottis phonatoria). Cs Otolaryng 30:28–31

Sisson GA (1980) Pseudoglottis procedure: update and secondary reconstruction techniques. The Laryngoscope 90:1120–1129

Staffieri M (1980) New surgical approaches for speech rehabilitation after total laryngectomy. In: Shedd DP, Weinberg B (eds) Surgical and prosthetic approaches to speech rehabilitation, pp 77–117

Steiner W (1980) Chirurgische Rehabilitation der Stimme nach Laryngektomie (derzeitiger Stand). Therapeutische Umschau 37/12:1117–1127

Tiwari RM (1982) Observations on surgical rehabilitation of voice after laryngectomy with Staffieri's method. J Laryng Otol 91:241–250

Tiwari RM (1982) Observations on surgical restoration of voice after laryngectomy. Ind J Otolaryngol 34:6–8

Vuyk HD (1984) Role of the upper esophageal sphincter in voice rehabilitation after laryngectomy and Staffieri procedure

Amatsu's Technique Using the Blom-Singer Tracheostoma Valve

M. AMATSU, K. MAKINO, M. KINISHI, M. TANI and M. KOKUBU[1]

For more than 20 years, various surgical techniques for postlaryngectomy voice restoration have been described. To create voice in the laryngectomized gullet, the trachea should be connected to the pharynx or oesophagus by a tract so that the diverted exhaled pulmonary air vibrates the gullet wall. The tract, however, always carries the potential risk of allowing dietary liquid to leak into the trachea. It is clear to see how a surgically-created tract without any sphincteric function or valve mechanism to close automatically during deglutition may allow liquid to leak from the gullet into the trachea.

Since we began a one-stage surgical technique for postlaryngectomy voice rehabilitation in 1976 (Amatsu 1977), our aim has been how to eliminate postoperative liquid aspiration completely. Another problem is the patient's having to use a finger to cover the tracheal opening so as to divert exhaled air into the oesophagus during phonation.

This paper describes a simple modification of the original technique using bilateral oesophageal muscle flaps in order to eliminate aspiration. It also includes our experiences with the Blom-Singer tracheostoma valve to eliminate finger use.

Techniques

The essential part of this technique consists in the construction of a tracheo-oesophageal speaking fistula using the membraneous part of the trachea (Amatsu 1978, 1980). If there is no suspicion of a subglottic extension, the larynx is removed just below the cricoid cartilage. The antero-lateral wall of the trachea is resected above the fifth tracheal ring in order to obtain an inferiorly-based tracheal flap while mainly using the membraneous part. The remaining cartilage on both margins of the tracheal flap is removed carefully by scissor dissection. The minimum length of the flap is 2.5 cm.

First, the lower half of the tracheostoma is formed and then a 1 cm midline vertical incision is made starting just below the superior margin of the tracheal flap entering the oesophageal lumen. A side-to-side anastomosis is created by approximating both incised mucosal margins of the membraneous trachea and

[1] Department of Otolaryngology, Kobe University Hospital, Kusmoki-cho, Chuo-ku, Kobe 650, Japan.

Speech Restoration Via Voice Prostheses
Edited by I. F. Herrmann

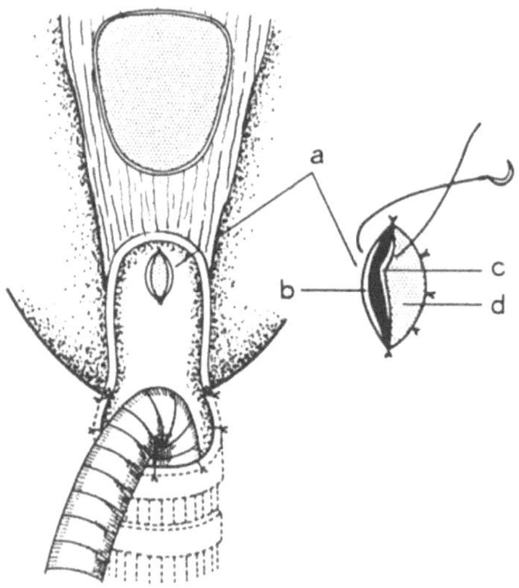

Fig. 1

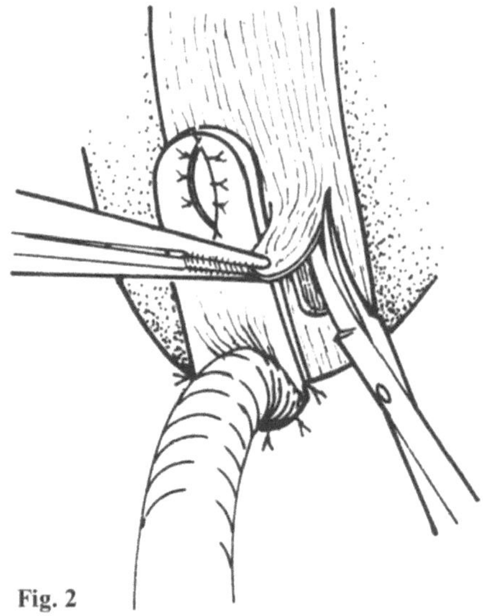

Fig. 2

Fig. 1. Creation of the oesophageal orifice of the shunt (side-to-side anastomosis). *a*, Oesophageal orifice of the shunt, *b*, tracheal mucosa, *c*, oesophageal mucosa, *d*, oesophageal lumen

Fig. 2. Oesophageal muscle flap (7 mm × 15 mm)

oesophagus with 8 stitches of 4-0 chromic cat gut (Fig. 1). Special care should be taken to avoid a postoperative stenosis at this site by fine suturing.

After the oesophageal wall at the level of the tracheal flap has been exposed bilaterally by elevating the inferior pole of the thyroid gland using blunt dissection, a superiorly-based oesophageal muscle flap is obtained which includes both the inner and outer muscle layers (7 mm × 15 mm) (Fig. 2). The base of this flap should not go beyond the level of the side-to-side anastomosis. It is important not to perforate the oesophageal mucosa.

The hypopharyngeal defect is closed by a horizontal line which meets the vertical line in a "T" fashion. To facilitate postoperative phonation, the hypopharyngeal muscle layers are left unsutured. After a 12th Fr. rubber catheter has been inserted upwards through the side-to-side anastomosis into the pharynx, both the lateral margins of the tracheal flap are approximated from above with 4-0 chromic catgut. This creates a mucosal-lined tube connecting the upper cervical oesophagus with the tracheostoma (Fig. 3).

After the construction of the mucosal tube, bilateral oesophageal muscle flaps are approximated with 3 stitches of 4-0 chromic catgut over the middle level of the tracheo-oesophageal shunt (Fig. 4).

Thyroid glands are replaced so as to eliminate dead space. They must be anchored to the neighboring structure, if necessary. The upper half of the tracheostoma is formed and the skin incision then closed. The rubber catheter in the shunt is anchored to the chest-wall for two weeks after surgery.

Speech can be produced by occlusion of the tracheostoma which diverts the exhaled air into the oesophagus.

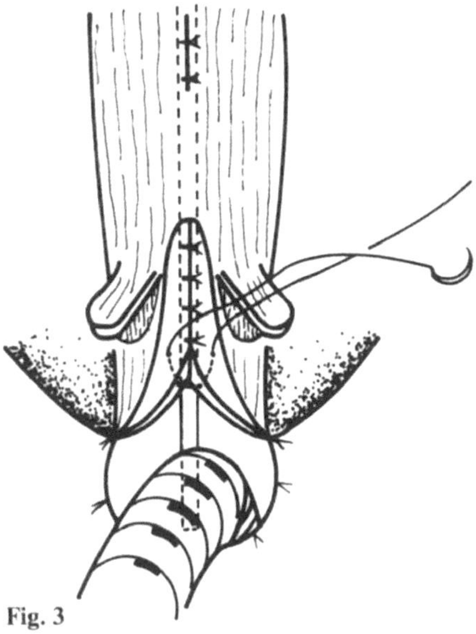

Fig. 3

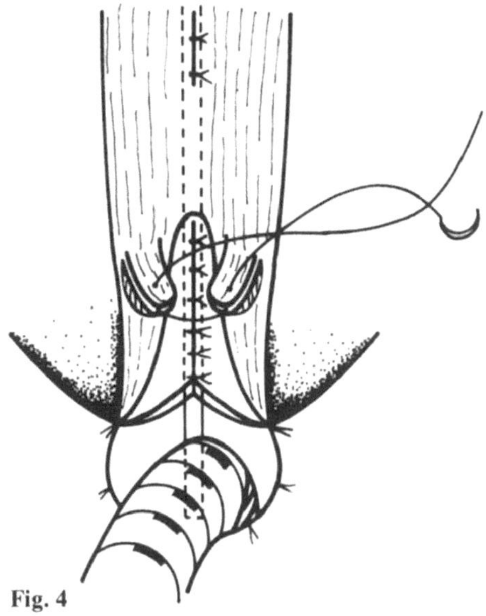

Fig. 4

Fig. 3. Construction of the tracheo-oesophageal shunt by approximating both lateral margins of the tracheal flap

Fig. 4. Bilateral oesophageal muscle flaps are approximated over the middle level of the tracheo-oesophageal shunt with 3 stitches of 4-0 chromic catgut

Results

We were encouraged by both postoperative phonatory function and deglutition without aspiration when using this technique. 10 patients were operated on with this technique. Of these patients, 9 were male and 1 was female. Their ages ranged from 32 years to 71 years. The data are listed in summarized form in Table 1.

Table 1. Summary of data

No.	Age and Sex	Tumour	Neck dissection	Radiation (preop. rad)	Phonation time (s)	Remarks
1	56 m	gl.	–	6,000	21	
2	42 m	supra.	unilat.	4,000	40	
3	39 f	supra.	bilat.	4,000	18	
4	63 m	gl.	–	6,000	34	
5	68 m	gl.	–	6,000	30	
6	32 m	supra.	–	7,000	25	
7	67 m	supra.	–	–	–	Blom-Singer prosthesis
8	60 m	supra.	unilat.	–		oesophageal speech
9	71 m	supra.	unilat.	–	15	
10	57 m	supra.	unilat.	–	10	

m, male; f, female

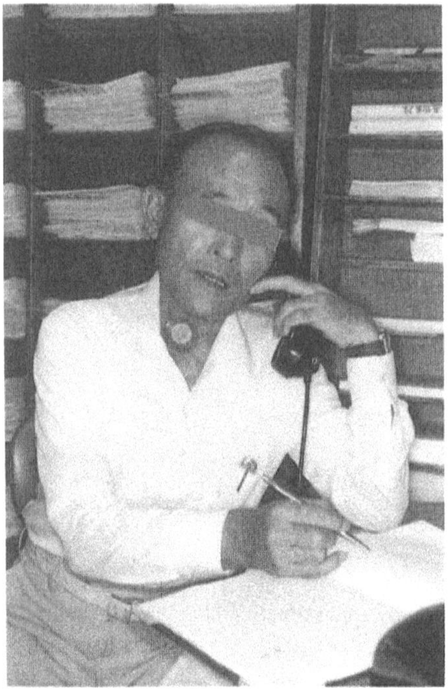

Fig. 5. A patient speaking with the Blom-Singer tracheostoma valve without manual occlusion of the stoma during speech

8 patients attained excellent speech ability. Deglutition was quite satisfactory. No aspiration occurred at all in these patients. 2 patients failed to speak with the shunt due to stenosis. Of these 2 patients, 1 underwent an endoscopic puncture (Singer and Blom 1980) for prosthesis speech and attained satisfactory speech ability and the other developed oesophageal speech spontaneously. In the latter patient, tracheo-oesophageal speech was attained by frequent dilation with a bougie for 2 months postoperatively but lasted only 2 days after that. During the above period, the patient learned to speak proficiently by vibrating the oesophageal wall with exhaled pulmonary air and did not require any oesophageal speech training.

A postoperative barium study revealed the sphincteric function of the shunt. Aspiration is avoided because the shunt is compressed from behind by the dilated oesophagus during swallowing, while the oesophageal flaps, approximated just in front of the shunt, do not allow it to move forwards.

In 6 of the 8 shunt speakers, the Blom-Singer tracheostoma valve (Blom et al. 1982) eliminated manual occlusion of the stoma during speech (Fig. 5). The other 2 shunt speakers found it difficult to use the valve because it could slip from place when the housing tape seal loosened. This was due to back pressure on the stoma during speech production.

Discussion

The advantages of the surgical techniques described above are:
1. no compromise with laryngectomy
2. safety
3. simplicity
4. one-stage, and 5. excellent postoperative speech ability.

The disadvantages are:
1. possible risk of aspiration (with dietary liquid only), and
2. use of finger for phonation.

There is no doubt that any form of tract between the trachea and gullet enables the laryngectomee to attain excellent speech ability. However, as has been mentioned, there is also no doubt that the tract induces aspiration without a sphincteric function or valve mechanism to allow air only to pass from the trachea into gullet for phonation.

The only possible way of preventing aspiration accompanying presentday voice restoration techniques is to use a prosthesis with a valve mechanism. The use of the oesophageal flaps described here could eliminate aspiration without reducing speech ability. Barium studies revealed that sphincteric function prevented aspiration.

6 patients in this series felt much more comfortable using the Blom-Singer tracheostoma valve than with manual occlusion of the stoma. As previously described (Blom et al. 1982), both excessive pharyngeal tone and even shunt resistance itself seemed to be related to difficulties in using the valve for 2 shunt speakers.

Summary

A recent modification of the original tracheo-oesophageal shunt operation described in this report eliminates the problem of aspiration completely. This newer technique, in combination with the use of the Blom-Singer tracheostoma valve, enables the laryngectomee to return to a near normal daily life.

References

Amatsu M (1978) A new one stage surgical technique for postlaryngectomy speech. Arch Otorhinolaryngol 220:149–152

Amatsu M (1980) A one-stage technique for postlaryngectomy voice rehabilitation. Laryngoscope 90:1378–1386

Amatsu M et al. (1977) Vocal rehabilitation after total laryngectomy – a new one-stage surgical technique –. Jap Jour Otol Tokyo 80:779–785

Blom ED et al. (1982) Tracheostoma valve for postlaryngectomy voice rehabilitation. Ann Otol Rhinol Laryngol 91:576–578

Singer MI, Blom ED (1980) An endoscopic technique for restoration of voice after laryngectomy. Ann Otol Rhinol Larnygol 89:529–533

Fingerless Voice Restoration Using Amatsu's Technique

H. RUDERT[1]

In 1979 I reported my first experiences with the voice rehabilitative laryngectomies of Staffieri and Amatsu. Besides aspiration, one of the disadvantages is that the tracheostoma has to be closed with a finger for voice production. There follows a report on one particular patient who learned to speak without using a finger.

A 52 year old male patient was laryngectomized in 1978. During the operation, a tracheo-oesophageal shunt was constructed according to Amatsu's technique. The patient, a manager by profession, learned to speak very quickly and only had a few problems with aspiration. However, he was angry that he had no hand free for writing when speaking on the telephone. Two years after the oper-

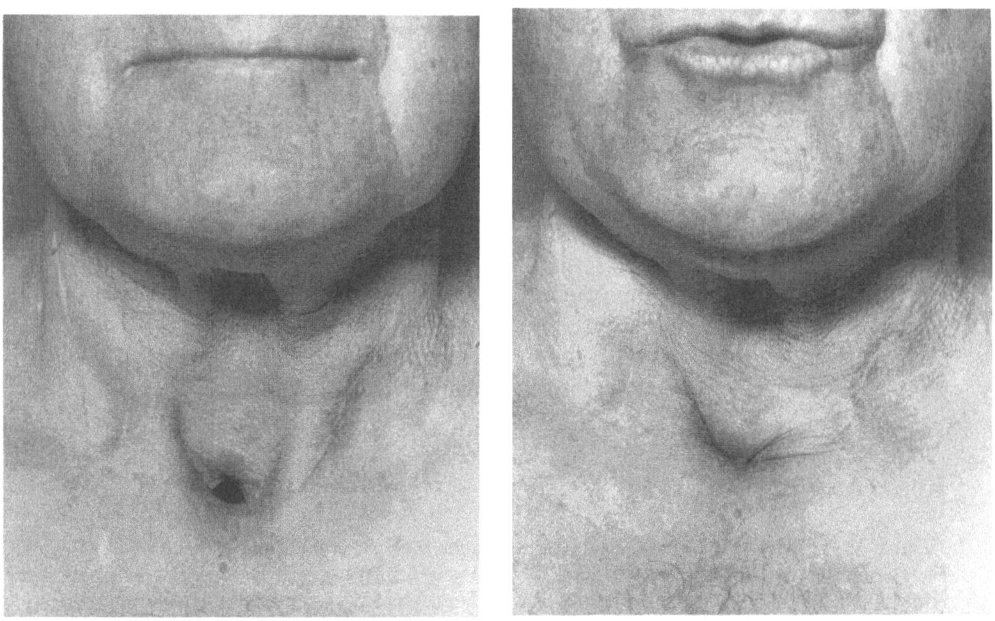

Figs. 1 a, b. Tracheostoma after voice rehabilitative laryngectomy (Amatsu's technique). **a** Tracheostoma in respiration, **b** tracheostoma closed by active contraction of the platysma muscle while speaking

[1] Klinik und Poliklinik für Hals-, Nasen- und Ohrenkrankheiten der Universität Kiel, Hospitalstraße 20, D-2300 Kiel.

Speech Restoration Via Voice Prostheses
Edited by I. F. Herrmann

ation, he visited me and spoke to me without using a finger. He had learned to close his tracheal stoma by the active contraction of his platysma muscle.

This man tolerates the discomfort of occasional aspiration. Unfortunately, this technique was not reproducible. It is hoped, however, that this example might provide the impulse to create a new technique. It ought to be possible to construct a sphincter with platysma muscle, which closes the tracheostoma by voluntary innervation.

References

Amatsu M (1978) A new one-stage surgical technique for postlaryngectomy speech. Arch Otorhinolaryng 220:149–152

Rudert H (1979) Erste Erfahrungen mit den Shunt-Operationen nach Staffieri und Amatsu. Zur Rehabilitation der Stimme nach Laryngektomie. Laryng Rhinol 58:476–481

Staffieri M (1973) Funktionelle total Laryngektomie (Chirurgische Technik, Indikation und Resultate einer eigenen Technik zur Glottisplastik mt Wiederherstellung der Stimme). Mschr Ohrenheilkunde (Wien) 107:77–89

Experience with the ESKA-Herrmann Tracheostoma Valve

I. F. Herrmann[1] and W. Koss[2]

Introduction

Not only voice loss but also the existence of a permanent tracheostoma are severe handicaps after laryngectomy. We should therefore try to achieve:

a) Intelligible fluent speech with good modulation, no aspiration, and no finger to close the tracheostoma.
b) The reconstruction of the respiratory tract without a permanent tracheostoma.

Part of the first aim can be achieved by glottoplasty with functional pharynx surgery and tracheostomaplasty. This method enables voice rehabilitation with low phonatory pressure, good voice modulation, and a tracheostoma in which a tracheostoma valve can be fitted. The required surgical techniques are described in the chapter "Glottoplasty with Functional Pharynx Surgery and Tracheostomaplasty" (p. 116). One important factor for the social and professional reintegration of laryngectomees is the tracheostoma valve. These valves allow voice production without finger occlusion.

Blom and Singer have developed a tracheostoma valve which is stuck onto the skin of the neck: The flap valve is good. Different valve strengths are needed to vary valve sensitivity. The problem with this technique, however, is that tracheal secretion allows the tracheostoma valve to stick to the skin of the neck for only a few hours. We have developed a tracheostoma valve which eliminates this problem. The results of the experiments which helped to develop this tracheostoma valve have already been given.

The Instrumental Set

The tracheostoma stent is made up of a cannula part and 3 different types of outer silicon ring to retain the tracheostoma stent (Fig. 1). The stent itself is made of very soft silicon and has no magnet. The cannula part of the tracheostoma valve is identical in shape to the tracheostoma stent. The flap valve contains a metal piece located off centre and is controlled by a magnet fixed in the cannula part. The sensitivity of the tracheostoma valve can be adjusted to individual needs by turning the flap value.

[1] Universitätsklinik und Poliklinik für Hals-, Nasen- und Ohrenkranke im Kopfklinikum, D-8700 Würzburg.
[2] Industriestraße, D-6222 Geisenheim.

Speech Restoration Via Voice Prostheses
Edited by I. F. Herrmann

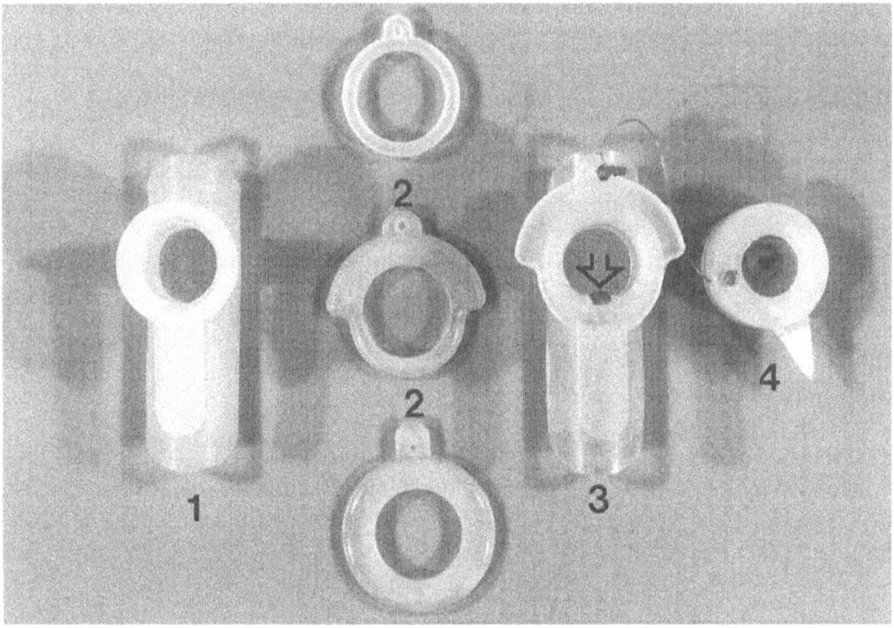

Fig. 1. *1*, The tracheostoma valve stent; *2*, three different retention collars; *3*, the tracheostoma cannula part of the tracheostoma valve with a permanent magnet (*arrow*); *4*, the flap valve

The Fitting and General Care of the Tracheostoma Valve (Fig. 2)

The tracheostoma stent is changed and cleaned on a daily basis. The tracheostoma valve is fitted 10–12 days after total laryngectomy once the dietary tube has been removed and the voice prosthesis inserted. The flap valve is then taken out

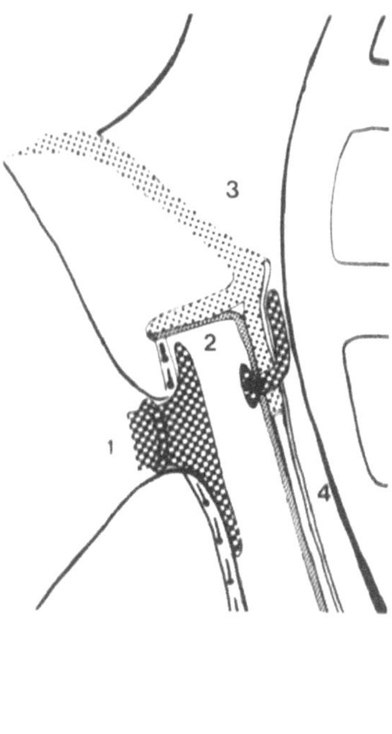

Fig. 2. *1*, The fitted tracheostoma valve; *2*, the tracheal chimney; *3*, the pharynx; *4*, the oesophagus

of the cannula and the tracheal mucosa around the tracheostoma locally anaesthetized. The cannula part of the tracheostoma valve is smeared with sliding gel. The patient holds his breath after expiring and the cannula part is gently inserted. If there is any play on the cannula part, it will not be airtight. A different or further silicon ring type can be drawn over to seal it. The tracheostoma valve is worn night and day. The tracheostoma valve can be cleaned without having to be changed. The average retention duration of the tracheostoma valve is up to 5 days. Wet skin or secretion do not affect its use. Speech is both easy and fluent if the voice prosthesis functions properly and the tracheostoma valve has been fitted correctly. No hands are needed.

Contra-Indications

Intense pulmonary emphysema, chronic recurrent (especially hypersecretory) bronchitis, feeble-mindedness, and alcoholism, are all contra-indications. At least one fully effective arm must be able to remove or replace the tracheostoma valve cannula or the flap valve.

Results

23 patients were fitted with a tracheostoma valve. Occasionally, the tracheostoma valve reduced the voice volume.

Reference

Blom ED, Singer MI, Hamaker RC (1982) Tracheostoma valve for postlaryngectomy voice rehabilitation. Ann Otol 91:576

Implantation of the Recurrent Nerve and Its Possible Use as a Trigger for an Artificial Larynx

I. F. HERRMANN [1]

The development of an artificial larynx requires the control of respiratory, vocal and coughing functions. The disadvantage of mechanical regulation is that the air flow and pressure resulting from physical exertion can almost equal voice insert values. This makes the valve close during the deep expiration phase. Such a problem would be solved if the respiratory valve could be successfully regulated by muscles acting on the stimulus of the recurrent nerve.

Method

During neck dissection, both portions of the sternocleidomastoid muscle near the sternum and clavicle are separated and transected so that the ends of the juxtaposed muscle stumps can be joined together later.

In the course of the laryngectomy, the recurrent nerve is prepared in its cervical position so that it can be split at the entrance to the larynx. After careful preparation of the nerve stump, it is fixed between the denervated muscle stumps of the sternocleidomastoid muscle by suturing the nerve to the muscle fibres. Both muscle stumps are then sutured around the nerve.

For the sake of comparison, the muscle stumps of 3 patients were sutured without implanting the recurrent nerve.

After the wound has healed, the muscle loop undergoes toning treatment for several weeks in order to prevent muscle degeneration.

Results

The recurrent nerve was implanted in seven patients; implantation was omitted in three cases. After three months, EMG tests were made to ascertain whether the sternocleidomastoid stumps had been reinnervated in all the patients (Fig. 1). A random spontaneous innervation was found to be possible. By contrast, no motor unit potentials were found in the muscular loop of the 3 patients who had not undergone nerve implantation. The sternocleidomastoid muscle was tensed by exerting pressure on the forehead (Fig. 2). Electrodes were placed in mirror-image

[1] Universitätsklinik und Poliklinik für Hals-, Nasen- und Ohrenkranke im Kopfklinikum, D-8700 Würzburg.

Speech Restoration Via Voice Prostheses
Edited by I. F. Herrmann

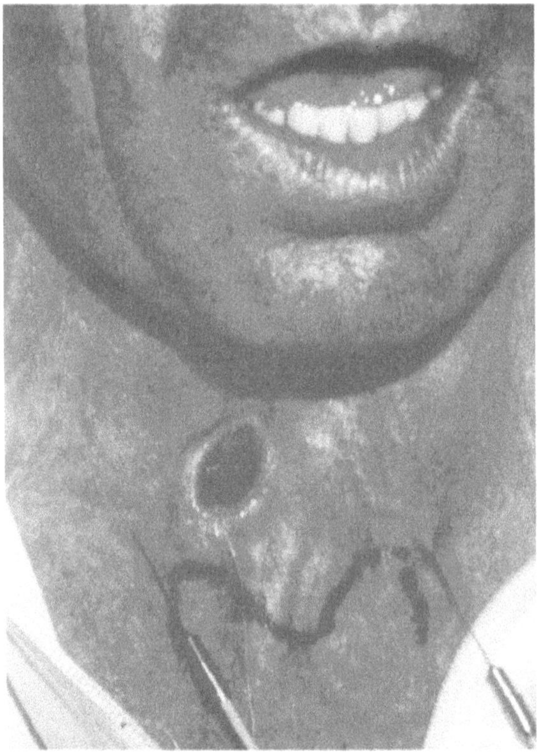

Fig. 1. EMG-registration during phonation

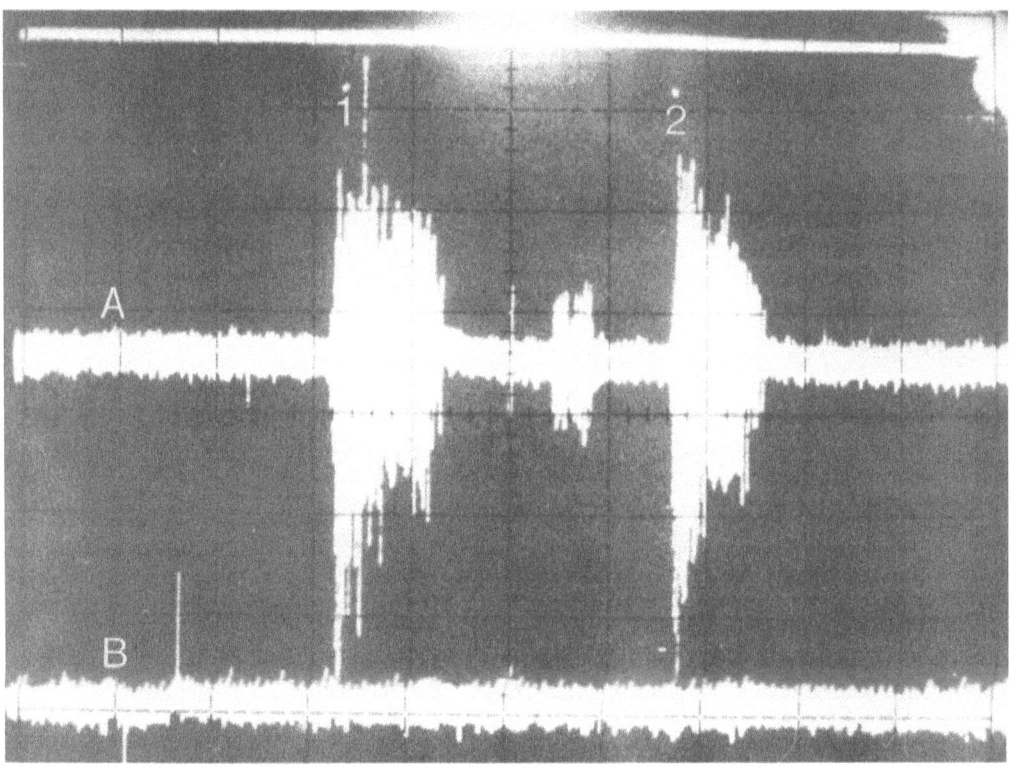

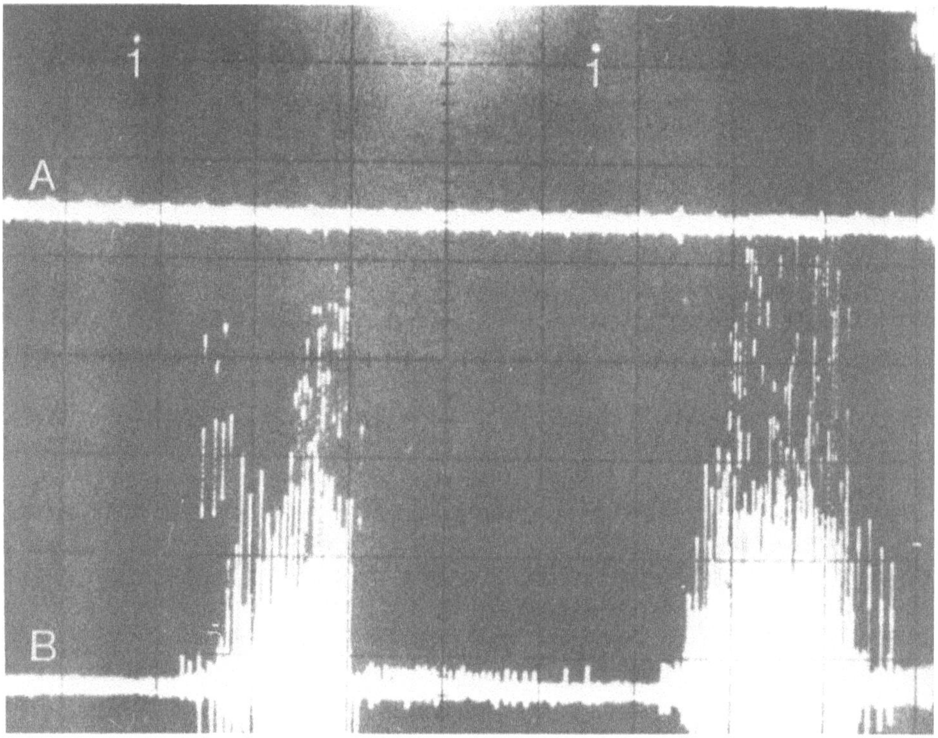

Fig. 3. EMG pattern during pressure on the forehead (1–1)

to each other on both sides of the throat. It was shown that muscle innervated by the accessory nerve was active. An EMG test was made on the muscle stumps connected to the recurrent nerve during phonation (Fig. 3).

Conclusion

The results show that after its reinnervation by recurrent nerve axons the muscle action potentials of the sternocleidomastoid muscle can be recorded. Recordings were made both in relation to respiration and phonation. They could be seen either alone or together for any given patient. As no EMG mirror-image recordings of the intact muscle could be found in the control group, muscle activity may well be triggered by the recurrent nerve.

Further research will try to develop a valve that can be activated by muscle potentials.

◀ **Fig. 2.** EMG pattern during phonation: *A*, sternocleidomastoid muscle stumps with nerve implantation (50 μV – 2 s/div); *B*, sternocleidomastoid muscle innervated by accessorius nerve (100 μV – 2 s/div); *1*, phonation "23"; *2*, phonation "A"

Chapter 8 Experimental Research to Establish an Artificial Larynx

Experimental Research to Establish an Artificial Larynx*

I. F. HERRMANN [1], C. HAMMER [2] and B. GREVEMEYER [2]

Introduction

Gluck (cited in Gottstein 1900) first introduced esophageal speech as a language restoration method for laryngectomy in 1882. He separated the respiratory and digestive tract and was able to achieve voice rehabilitation without aspiration for some of his patients. No radical improvements have since been made. The stigma of a permanent tracheostoma has never been removed.

We have successfully achieved voice rehabilitation regardless of tumor side or extension (Herrmann et al. 1984; Herrmann and Koss 1985). Fingerless speech is being tested. Previous work with the removal of the permanent tracheostoma has been unacceptably hindered by the necessity for radical tumor resection (Serafini 1974). Even attempted larynx transplants (Kluyskens and Ringoir 1970), which seemed to be promising at first, were later rejected for technical, immunological, tumor surgical and ethical reasons. Sixteen years have passed without any further ideas considering the removal of the permanent tracheostoma after laryngectomy.

Preliminary Remarks

Animal experiments with an artificial larynx must fulfill the following qualifications:

- Respiration without aspiration
- An artificial larynx must always be replacable as defects can cause dangerous respiratory problems.

Furthermore, surgical techniques must be developed which enable both primary insertion of an artificial larynx, which is done during laryngectomy, and a secondary insertion, which is sometimes years after the laryngectomy.

* Dedicated to Professor Dr. H. G. Boenninghaus, Heidelberg.

[1] Universitätsklinik und Poliklinik für Hals-, Nasen- und Ohrenkranke im Kopfklinikum, D-8700 Würzburg.
[2] Institut für chirurgische Forschung, Klinikum Großhadern, Marchioninistraße 15, D-8000 München 70.

Speech Restoration Via Voice Prostheses
Edited by I. F. Herrmann

Table 1. Prescription of the inhalation fluid

Tacholiquin (Tyloxapol)	50 ml
Bepanthen (Dexyanthenol)	50 ml
α-Chymotrase (α-Chymotrypsin)	10 ml
Refobacin (Gentamycin)	4 ml
Aqua bidest	ad 1000 ml

Material and Methods

Male baboons weighing over 20 kilogrammes were used: During quarantine and preparation time the animals received primate food and fruits as well as water ad libidum. These animals met the following criteria:

- Their trachea is wide enough to allow the implantation of an artificial larynx without impeding respiration.
- Their anatomy came nearest to that of human beings (position of the larynx, relationship in size between the larynx and the pharynx, relationship between the total neck length and cervical muscles etc.)
- They swallow in a partly upright position.

7 male baboons were laryngectomized over the last two years: 4 animals were subjected to a primary and 3 animals to a secondary insertion of an artificial larynx.

The usual surgical instruments were used for laryngectomy. Malfunctions caused by swallowing, followed by aspiration were prevented by filling the artificial larynx out with gaze. All animals were weighed and CBC (complete blood count) was submitted the day before surgery. The dressing was changed daily in the postoperative period and weight was determined under short anaesthesia. Feeding by tube was applied from the first day on after surgery. Enteral feeding followed the nutritional plan. Fresubine was supplied supplementary from the fifth day on. Depending on how much the animals ate, they were fed parenterally and through a stomach tube when they had their bandage changed only every 2 days until the 10th day.

It was regularly necessary to complement enteral with parenteral feeding as the animals lost weight after surgery. They were supplied electrolyte solutions, 10% glucose-solution, and aminoacids solution. The reconstruction needs to be non-stenotic and complete air tight to prevent subcutaneous emphysema. Tracheal stenosis as a result of postoperative granulation tissue formation is minimized by precise surgical technique, by use of minimally reactive absorbable suture material, and by gentle tissue handling. Infections, intraluminal suture materials and knots and such a line tension stimulate formation of granulation tissue.

Two ultrasound inhalators (Heyer et al.) were used to avoid inflammation of the respiratory tract. Tacholiquin (Tyloxapol), Bepanthen (Dexpanthenol), Alphachymotrase (Alphachymotrypsin), and Refobacin (Gentamycin) were added to the inhalation fluid (Table 1). The inhalators worked night and day during the period when the animals were tracheostomized.

Table 2. Anaesthesia

Premedication:	Ketantest (Ketamin) Parke Davis, München, FRG, 2,5 mg/kg i.m. Rompun (Xylazin) Bayer, Leverkusen, FRG, 1 mg/kg i.m.
Inhalation anesthetic:	Halothan (Halothan) Höchst, Frankfurt, FRG
Short intravenous narcosis:	used during bandage change Hypnomidate (Etomidat) Jonsen, Neuss, FRG, 0,2 mg/kg i.v.

Surgical Procedure

Anaesthesia: The animals were immobilized by using 1 ml Ketamin (2,5 mg/kg) and 1 mg/kg Xylazin. For operation N_2O/Halothananaesthesia was applied (Table 2).

1. Primary Insertion of an Artificial Larynx in a One Step Operation with the Laryngectomy

- The baboons neck is aseptically prepared.
- Surgical procedure:

Skin incision; preparation of the platysma fascia flap; blunt preparation and resection of the roar sac; skeletization of the larynx; lateral displacement of the thyroid glands; exposure and protection of the external branch of the bilateral cranial laryngeal nerves; separation of the thyreo-pharyngeal and crico-pharyngeal muscles at the thyroid and cricoid cartilage; resection of the larynx in standard fashion in the cause of which a caudally pediculated mucosal flap is cut from the paries membranaceus of the trachea (this volume, p. 116).

The ventral third of the third and fourth tracheal cartilage is excised and the mucosa is incised cruciformly. The tubus is then changed. Blunt mobilization of

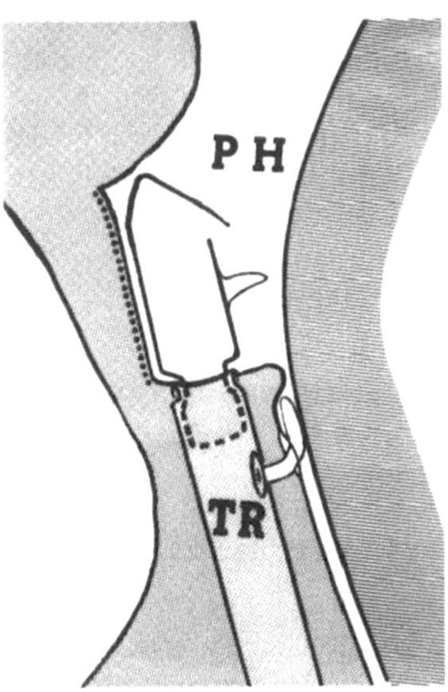

Fig. 1. Scheme: primary insertion of an artificial larynx. *PH*, Pharynx; *TR*, trachea

Table 3. Antibiotics

Tardomyocel Comp. III, Bayer Leverkusen	
200000 I.E.	Benzylpenicillin
50 mg	Procain-Benzylpenicillin
550 mg	Streptomycin

the pharynx while protecting the external branches of the cranial laryngeal nerve. Median myotomy of the oropharynx to the upper oesophagus. The dorsal muscle stumps of the pharyngeal constrictor muscle are pushed down bluntly to the side and then fixed to the prevertebral muscles paramedially using a continuous suture.

An everting tongue base flap is created by resecting a part of the tongue base muscle while preserving the lingual arteries. A suture is then made between the tongue base flap and the platysma fascia flap including the muscle originating from the hyoid (after resecting of the hyoid). This creates a wide pharynx. Exposure of the dorsal ends of the first tracheal cartilages and their fixation with two interrupted button sutures.

The trachea which is to be connected to the platysma fascia flap is drawn slightly cranially. The ventral pharynx wall is sewed along the median line at the cranial end of the trachea. The caudally pediculated mucosal flap of the posterior tracheal wall is sutured to the caudal part of the split pharyngeal wall. The lateral tracheal mucosa is also joined to the pharyngeal mucosa.

A piece of cartilage is resected from the anterior wall of the first tracheal ring. The artificial larynx is inserted into the cranial end of the trachea (Fig. 1). The gap in the first tracheal ring is then closed by suturing the ventral cartilage ends. The larynx is secured. The lateral pharyngeal walls are sutured to the platysma fascia flap (Herrmann 1984).

The tracheostoma is applied in the usual way once the pharynx has been closed. Hemostasis, careful stitching in the tracheostoma region, and bandaging are essential for proper cicatrization, especially as it is not possible to apply a Redon drainage on these animals. We overcome this problem by using fibrin tissue glue. Serom formation or emphysema usually cause serious complications.

The animals are given antibiotics for the first 8–10 days (Table 3).

2. Secondary Insertion of an Artificial Larynx After Laryngectomy

The surgical procedure is divided into three parts:

a) The laryngectomy with functional pharynx surgery and tracheostomaplasty as described in chapter an earlier chapter (see p. 116);
b) the positioning of the silicon stent, and
c) the insertion of the artificial larynx.

The aim of this procedure is to provide patients with an artificial larynx without tracheostoma years after the laryngectomy.

ad a. The laryngectomy basically follows the procedure described above. Muscle exzision in the area around the tongue base with application of a tongue base flap were also necessary in animal experiments. After hyoid resection a suture is made between the tongue base flap and the platysma fascia flap which includes the upper tongue bone muscle. This creates a wide pharynx. In addition, the posterior ends of the first tracheal cartilage ring are exposed and secured with two absorbable sutures. The postoperative care of the animals was identical to that described above.

ad b. A silicon stent is inserted 3–4 weeks after the laryngectomy between the cranial end of the trachea and the base of the tongue.

Surgical procedure: Incision in the scare; preparation of the skin flap; exposure of the sternal part of the sternocleidomastoid muscle; measurement of the muscle flap needed to cover the place retainer; creation of the muscle flap caudally hanged on a pedicle; exposure of the closed canal end of the trachea; fitting of the stent without injuring the trachea or pharyngeal wall; covering of the stent ventrally and laterally with a sternocleidomastoid muscle flap; suturing the muscle flap around the stent; subcutaneous suture; skin clamping. The stent is left inside for at least 3 weeks. Scar tissue formation around the silicon during this period and thereby ensures a tight close of the scar around the artificial larynx.

ad c. Surgical procedure: Reopening of the old scar with scar exzision; preparation of the skin flap; the muscle fibres of the sternocleidomastoid muscle are separated over the stent; the formed capsule is split and the stent extracted.

The first tracheal ring is exposed and split along the medial line. The hypopharynx is inspected with a strong oesophagoscope. The oesophagoscope is secured on the median line just below the base of the tongue so that it can serve as a base for the incision of the hypopharynx. The dorsal ends of the first tracheal ring were already secured by suturing during the first operation.

Opening of the tracheal roof above the first tracheal ring. The first ring is sewered. The artificial larynx is pushed gently by its rare incision into the first tra-

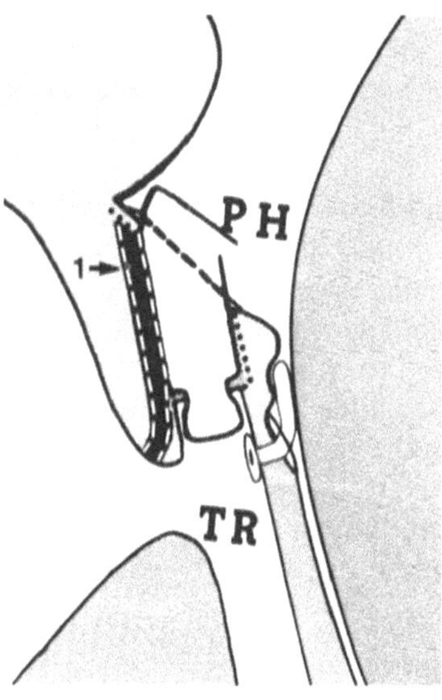

Fig. 2. Scheme: after the third part of secondary inserting an artificial larynx. *PH*, Pharynx; *TR*, trachea; *l*, musculus sternocleidomastoideus flap

cheal ring. The anterior end of the first tracheal cartilage move apart. A small piece is excised from the first tracheal ring, where necessary and the gap is closed by simple interrupted sutures. The capsule formed by the stent and the sternal part of the sternocleidomastoid muscle are then closed over the artificial larynx. Completing skin suture, treatment is the same as described in 1 (Fig. 2).

The oblique protective cover over the artificial larynx stops food and liquid from getting between the mucous membrane and the artificial larynx. The protective cover is closely attached to the mucous membrane.

Results

For our current prospective, the development of an artificial larynx was a numerous problem because of the baboons' high intelligence, their tearing and their wounds and inability to cooperate. This difficulties must be managed in future work with these animals.

The following serious problems occurred:

1. A cervical thorax plaster of Paris cast had to be used because the animals would otherwise tear at their tracheostoma and stitches.
2. As the tracheostoma remains for at least ten days after primary insertion and roughly 5 weeks after secondary insertion, there was always the risk of tracheal infection via external contamination despite excellent aftercare.
3. No research reports on the enteral and parenteral feeding of baboons exists. There is a risk of lung edema because feeding during the first 4 days after the operation is only possible under anaesthesia and larger weight losses have to be avoided as to ensure proper cicatrization. To reduce this risk oral feeding is done as soon as possible (i.e. 4th day after surgery).

Further problems were:

- the lack of exact anatomical data, e.g., regarding the size of the larynx, inner and outer diameter of the trachea, etc.,
- the lack of knowledge regarding longer-lasting anaesthetics on these animals,
- the danger of post-operative serom formation and tracheostoma infections with only one daily change of bandage,
- the impossibility of applying a suction draine,
- the difficulties encountered when applying venous feeds the 3rd or 4th day after the operation, etc.

Despite the above problems, increasing experience allowed the artificial larynx to heal in the last three animals and to let them live with an artificial larynx for up to 6 weeks. Both operative techniques proved to be satisfactory.

After only 14 days, the first tracheal ring was so stable that it was possible to change the artificial larynx twice without splitting the ring. The artificial larynx is changed endoscopically. During this procedure, the trachea has to be secured manually from the outside to prevent any movement of the respiratory tract when the artificial larynx is clipped in.

Discussion

Past attempts to rehabilitate laryngectomized patients have concentrated primarily on voice restoration. The tracheostoma has been accepted as a necessary evil without much debate. No attempts have been made specifically to avoid a tracheostoma.

Laryngectomies since Gluck have eliminated the joint stretch between the respiratory and digestive tracts in order to avoid aspiration. It could only be reconstructed if it were possible to adapt the stiff tracheal tube to the flexible digestive tract by means of an artificial larynx with nonaspiration and sufficient respiration. However, a primary larynx transplant is not safe enough to be justified because the main aim of every laryngectomy is the complete and safe removal of a tumor and the necessary immunosuppression would reduce endogenous defence against any remaining tumor cells. A transplant is therefore only acceptable at least 2–3 years after the operation with a high probability of tumor freedom for the patient. Even this secondary process will only be worth discussing if the next 2 or 3 years allow the development of a suitable larynx substitute.

The main requirement for any new artificial larynx is ease of change as functional impairment can be perilous. Basically, there are two ways in which it can be fixed.

One way is to implant a foundation structure above and around the trachea to which the artificial larynx is then connected. However, the healing process can

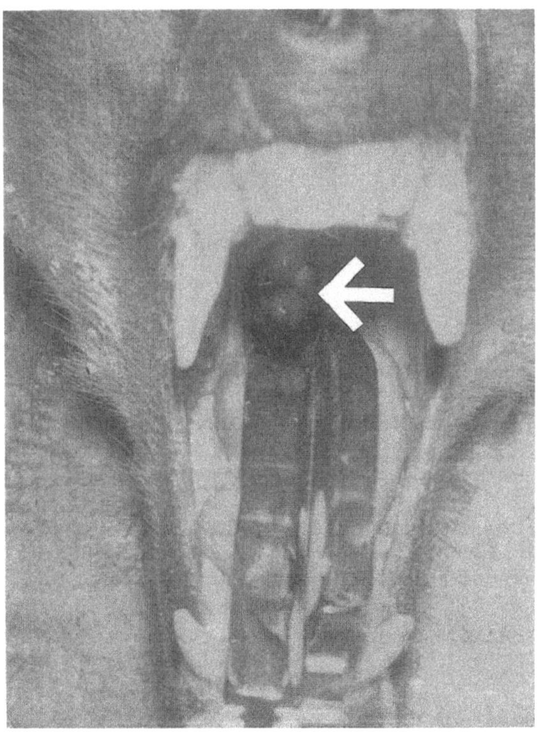

Fig. 3. Artificial larynx in situ (*arrow*)

often be impeded in the transition area between the implant and the larynx connection.

The other way of achieving complete ease of change is to fit the larynx into the trachea without prior implantation. In this case, larynx fixation requires surgery. We have thought of one possibility where the artificial larynx can be anchored by a rear incision in the region of the first intact tracheal ring.

If the larynx is inserted into the pharynx, the pharyngeal lumen must be sufficient enough to allow food intake alongside the larynx. In contrast to previous laryngectomy techniques, this means that the whole width of the oesophagus must be preserved. The area must be reconstructed where the inlet of the larynx opens into the pharynx together with the epiglottis, aryepiglottidian folds, arytenoid protuberance, interarytenoid region, and postcricoidal-situated mucous membrane. Only then is food intake possible without any risk of aspiration. This reconstruction was achieved by the development of a platysma fascia flap which truly enabled the creation of a wide pharyngeal lumen.

If the defect caused by a laryngectomy is to be reconstructed with a well-proportioned platysma fascia flap, a safety loop should be attached to the artificial larynx so as to avoid any danger of aspiration. This is because the flap has a known tendency to shrink (Herrmann 1984) and because of the contractility of the oesophagus. Food must be prevented from being pressed into the artificial larynx. Dorsomedian myotomy must also preserved innervation so as to guarantee the necessary peristalsis above and below the aspiration prevention ring. Experience has also been gained with the secondary insertion of an artificial larynx. It has been found that an artificial larynx can be inserted in a several stage operation some months after the laryngectomy under the above-mentioned conditions (Fig. 3).

Past experience allows it to be said that an artificial larynx can be made which is also easy to change. Its construction is currently under development.

Finally, many questions raised in this book still remain open. However, it has been the purpose of this book to pave the way towards new answers in our field of research.

References

Gottstein C (1900) Die Pseudostimme nach Totalexstirpation des Larynx. Arch Klin Chir 62:126

Herrmann IF (1984) Die Pharynxrekonstruktion mit dem Platysma-Faszienlappen. Laryng Rhinol Otol 63:274–276

Herrmann IF, Koss W (1985) Die fingerfreie Sprache nach totaler Laryngektomie. HNO 33:124–129

Herrmann IF, Buchwald J, Zenner HP (1984) Die Glottoplastik – eine neue Methode zur chirurgischen Stimmrehabilitation. HNO 32:294–301

Kluyskens P, Ringoir S (1970) Follow-up of a human larynx transplantation. Laryngoscope 80:1244–1250

Serafini I (1974) Laringectomia con anastomosi tracheofaringea. Tumori 60:531–546

Subject Index